The Benefits of Vitamins

POOJA BAJAJ MALHOTRA

NEW DAWN PRESS, INC.
USA• UK• INDIA

NEW DAWN PRESS GROUP

Published by New Dawn Press Group
New Dawn Press, Inc., 244 South Randall Rd # 90, Elgin, IL 60123
e-mail: sales@newdawnpress.com

New Dawn Press, 2 Tintern Close, Slough, Berkshire, SL1-2TB, UK
e-mail: sterlingdis@yahoo.co.uk

New Dawn Press (An Imprint of Sterling Publishers (P) Ltd.)
A-59, Okhla Industrial Area, Phase-II, New Delhi-110020
e-mail: sterlingpublishers@airtelbroadband.in
www.sterlingpublishers.com

The Benefits of Vitamins
© 2006, Pooja Bajaj Malhotra
ISBN 1 84557 645 4

All rights are reserved. No part of this publication may be reproduced, stored in a retrieval system or transmitted, in any form or by any means, mechanical, photocopying, recording or otherwise, without prior written permission of the publisher.

PRINTED IN INDIA

Contents

Introduction	5
Fat-soluble Vitamins	10
Vitamin A	12
Vitamin D	21
Vitamin E	29
Vitamin K	38
Water-soluble Vitamins	47
Thiamin	50
Riboflavin	57
Niacin	63
Vitamin B_6	71
Pantothenic Acid	80
Biotin	85
Folic Acid	91
Vitamin B_{12}	98
Vitamin C	105
Myths and Facts	113

Appendix I	Recommended Dietary Allowances	116
Appendix II	Vitamin Content of Common Foods	117

Introduction

Vitamins: The miracle workers

Welcome to the world of vitamins. The story of vitamins, their discovery, functions in maintaining health, and usefulness in healing deficiency diseases is fascinating. The term *'vitamins'* was first coined in the year 1912 by Casimir Funk, a Polish chemist. The first vitamin discovered was an amine. Since the substance discovered had life-giving properties, it was described as a 'vital amine' or 'vitamine'. The 'e' was later dropped because the substance was found to be a group of essential compounds, not all of which were amines.

Vitamins are not food but they are chemicals contained in food. They furnish no energy or building materials for the body. They participate in processes that are vital for health and normal body functions.

Vitamins is the name given to a group of potent organic compounds, other than protein, carbohydrate and fat, that are essential in minute quantities for specific body functions of growth, maintenance and reproduction. Vitamins regulate the chemical reactions by which the body utilises carbohydrates, proteins and fats to provide energy to the living tissues. They help in formation of blood cells, hormones, nervous system chemicals known as neurotransmitters, and the genetic material Deoxyribonucleic Acid (DNA).

There are about thirteen well-identified vitamins. Some vitamins are soluble in fat but not in water and vice-versa. Accordingly, they are classified as fat-soluble and water-soluble vitamins. Fat-soluble vitamins include vitamins A, D, E and K. These vitamins are generally present in foods containing fat. When fat is digested in the body, the fat-soluble vitamins are absorbed along with the breakdown products of fat digestion. Excess amounts of fat-soluble vitamins are stored in the body's fat deposits, liver and kidneys. Because the body stores fat-soluble vitamins, they can be eaten in large amounts once in a while and still meet the body's needs over a period of time. However, if fat-soluble vitamins are regularly consumed in very large amounts, they can reach dangerous levels producing toxic effects.

Water-soluble vitamins include vitamin C and the B complex vitamins comprising B_1 (thiamin), B_2 (riboflavin), B_3 (niacin), B_6 (pyridoxine), pantothenic acid, biotin, folic acid and B_{12} (cyanocobalamin).

Water-soluble vitamins are directly absorbed into the blood stream and travel freely in the blood. However, they cannot be stored and rapidly leave the body in the form of urine, if taken in greater quantities than the body can use. Water-soluble vitamins are retained in the body for varying periods of time. A single day's omission from the diet doesn't produce deficiency symptoms, but still, water-soluble vitamins must be eaten more regularly than fat-soluble vitamins.

Of the vitamins listed above, biotin, niacin, pantothenic acid, vitamin D and vitamin K are produced by our body in variable amounts. Only biotin, pantothenic acid and vitamin K, which are produced by bacteria in the human intestine, are possibly produced in sufficient quantities to meet the body's needs.

In addition to some of the roles of vitamins mentioned above, vitamins A, C and E function as antioxidants, which are vital in countering the potential harm of chemicals known as free radicals. If these free radicals remain unchecked, they can make cells more vulnerable to cancer-causing substances. Free radicals can also transform chemicals in the body to cancer-causing agents. Environmental pollutants, such as cigarette smoke, are sources of free radicals. An antioxidant is a substance that prevents the oxidation of another substance. In doing so, the antioxidant gets oxidized itself.

Each vitamin has such specific uses that one cannot replace, or act for, another. But the lack of one vitamin can interfere with the function of another. The continued lack of one vitamin in an otherwise complete diet results in vitamin deficiency diseases like beriberi, pellagra, rickets or scurvy. Most of the vitamins got discovered when scientists were searching for the causes of such diseases.

The best way to obtain vitamins is to eat a balanced diet that includes a variety of foods such as cereals, pulses, non-vegetarian foods, vegetables, fruits, sugars and fat, that provide an adequate supply of all the vitamins. A Recommended Dietary Allowance (RDA) has been established for most vitamins. The complete summary of dietary allowances for various nutrients as recommended by Indian Council Medical Research, ICMR, is given in Appendix I.

Almost all foods consumed by man are cooked, with the exception of fruits and some vegetables which are used for salads and chutneys. Cooking has both adverse and beneficial effects. The loss of nutrients during cooking depends on the temperature of cooking, duration of cooking and the nutrients present. Precooking practices such as cutting and washing also influence loss of nutrients. For example, cutting vegetables into small pieces and exposing them to air before cooking may result in loss of vitamins, particularly vitamin C. Washing and boiling of rice in excess water which is later discarded, also results in loss of vitamins and minerals. Vitamins of the water-soluble group are particularly susceptible to losses during cooking. With some precautions, however, the losses can be minimised. On the other hand, cooking is beneficial as it destroys harmful food-borne microorganisms. Some culinary practices such as fermentation in fact improve the nutritive value of foods.

Some health conscious people take vitamin supplements daily, in the form of tablets. These supplements contain one or more vitamins in the range of their RDAs. But a person who eats a balanced diet has no need for daily supplements. A person with a vitamin deficiency disease may take large doses of a certain vitamin or of a combination of vitamins under the guidance of a physician. Self-diagnosis and treatment with mega-doses (doses 10 or more times larger than the RDA) can be dangerous.

The following chapters will cover all the major vitamins, their functions in the body, their RDA, important food sources, and consequences of deficiency and excess. Appendix II gives the vitamin content of commonly consumed foods.

Fat-soluble Vitamins

Most of the vitamins were discovered from the years 1900 to 1950. It was found that a fat-soluble factor prevented xerophthalmia (dry eye disease) in rats, and the discoverers called it fat-soluble A factor. This factor is now known as vitamin A or retinol. Soon other fat-soluble factors (the fat-soluble vitamins A, D, E and K) were discovered.

Although the four fat-soluble vitamins (A, D, E and K) differ in function, utilisation, and sources, they also have several similar characteristics. They are soluble in fat and fat solvents; are fairly stable to heat, as in cooking; do not contain nitrogen; are absorbed in the intestine along with fat and lipids in foods; and require bile (greenish brown liquid to help the body to deal with fats) for absorption.

The fat-soluble vitamins A, D, E and K differ from the water-soluble vitamins in several ways. The fat-soluble vitamins are found in the fats and oils of food. They are insoluble in water, so they require bile for absorption. The fat-soluble vitamins are stored in the liver and adipose tissue (fatty tissue) until they are needed. They are not readily excreted from the body as most of the water-soluble vitamins are. Vitamins A and D are stored in large amounts for long periods of time and need not be consumed everyday. A person only needs to ensure that their average daily intake should be close to the recommended amount. Because the fat-soluble vitamins can be stored in the body, the risk of toxicity in case of fat-soluble vitamins is greater than it is for the water-soluble vitamins.

Vitamin A

Vitamin A was the first fat-soluble vitamin to be discovered by McCollum and Davis in 1913. Three different forms of vitamin A are active in the body: retinol, retinal and retinoic acid. Collectively, these are known as retinoid. In the natural form, retinoids are found only in animal foods, usually associated with lipids.

The original source of retinoids is the class of plant pigments known as carotenoids, which includes alpha, beta and gamma carotenes. These pigments were so called because one of their main source was carrot. Since carotenes can be converted to vitamin A in the body, they are often referred to as precursors of vitamin A or provitamin A. The main source of carotenes are dark green, leafy vegetables and yellow, orange and red fruits and vegetables.

Of all the carotenoids, betacarotene is the most plentiful in human foods. Carotenes are split in the intestine to form retinal which is then converted to retinol. Retinol is absorbed from the intestine and transported to the liver for storage. About 90% of body stores of vitamin A are found in the liver, the remaining stores are in the kidney, lungs, adrenal glands and adipose tissue. From the liver, vitamin A is transported to other tissues to be used for various body functions. A healthy adult has reserves of vitamin A that can last him for months.

Since the efficiency of conversion of betacarotene to retinol is not complete and absorption of carotenes is only about 50%, betacarotene is considered only one-fourth as effective as retinol on a weight-for-weight basis.

Vitamin A is soluble in fat and fat solvents but it is insoluble in water. Also, it is relatively stable to heat. Because of these reasons, vitamin A is fairly stable in general cooking.

Functions of vitamin A

Vitamin A is a versatile vitamin. Its major roles include:
- Promoting vision
- Participating in protein synthesis and cell differentiation (and thus it maintains the health of epithelial tissues and skin)
- Supporting reproduction and growth

Each form of vitamin A performs specific tasks. Retinol supports reproduction and is the major form in which the vitamin is transported and stored. Retinal actively helps in the betterment of the vision. Retinoic acid acts like a hormone, regulating cell differentiation, growth, and embryonic development.

Vitamin A in vision

Vitamin A plays an indispensable role. It participates in the conversion of light energy into nerve impulses at the retina of the eye, enabling us to see. Light passes through the cornea of the eye and strikes the cells of the retina. Inside the cells, pigment molecules called *rhodopsin* absorb light. Each rhodopsin molecule is composed of a protein called *opsin* and a molecule of retinal. When light energy strikes the retina, the configuration of the retinal changes and gets released from the rhodopsin molecule. This results in the generation of an electrical impulse, which is transmitted to the nerve cells which, in turn, convey the message to the brain. The released retinal has a different configuration and hence, it is inactive. Much of the retinal is converted back to its active form and combined with opsin to regenerate rhodopsin. A lot of retinal is destroyed at night and needs to be replenished through a good diet.

Vitamin A in protein synthesis and cell differentiation

Vitamin A participates in protein synthesis and cell differentiation. All body surfaces, both inside and outside, are covered by layers of epithelial cells. The epithelial tissue on the outside of the body is in the form of skin and those that line the inside of the body are the mucous membranes – the linings of the mouth, stomach, intestines, lungs, urinary bladder, urethra, uterus, vagina and so on. The epithelial tissue forms the first line of defence against invading microorganisms and infections. Vitamin A helps to maintain a healthy epithelium. It is also required for cell differentiation (development of specific functions) of bone, nerve and epithelial tissues.

Vitamin A in reproduction and growth
Vitamin A supports reproduction and growth. Retinol helps in sperm development in men and Vitamin A supports normal foetus development in women during pregnancy. Deficiency of vitamin A results in growth failure in children.

Betacarotene as an antioxidant
The provitamin A betacarotene has been shown to have antioxidant capacity, that is, it has the ability to protect a person against cell damage caused by free radicals. Free radicals are either parts of by-products of normal metabolism, or they may be created by environmental exposure to sunlight, tobacco smoke, car exhaust fumes, ozone, or x-rays. Free radicals damage the DNA,

cell membranes, and cell compounds, or even kill the cell. Antioxidant substances help neutralise free radicals in the cell, protecting the individual from possible damages.

Daily allowances of vitamin A

ICMR has established allowances of various nutrients for Indian population as per age, sex, activity status and other conditions. Table 1 contains the recommended daily allowances of vitamin A for all age groups and conditions.

Table 1
Recommended intake of vitamin A (mg/day)

Group	Retinol	Betacarotene
Adult men and women	600	2400
Pregnant women	600	2400
Lactating women	950	3800
Infants 0-12 months	35	1400
Preschool children 1-6 years	400	160
School children 7-12 years	600	2400
Adolescents 13-18 years	600	2400

Rich sources of vitamin A

Preformed vitamin A occurs only in foods of animal origin – liver, fish liver oils, egg, milk and milk products like cheese, butter, ghee, etc. Plant foods contain no preformed vitamin A, but many vegetables and fruits contain vitamin A precursors called carotenoids. Carotenes form the principle source of vitamin A in the diet and they are widespread in those plant foods that have high green, yellow, orange or red colour. The dark green leafy vegetables contain abundant amounts of the green pigment chlorophyll, which masks the yellow colour of the carotenes in them. Abundant sources of carotene are found in foods such as green leafy vegetables like spinach, turnip greens, beet greens, amaranth, coriander leaves, fenugreek leaves, mustard leaves and mint; yellow vegetables like carrot and pumpkin and yellow fruits like apricots, mango, orange, papaya; and raspberry.

An exhaustive list of vitamin content of all commonly consumed foods is given in Appendix II. Absence of data for any of the vitamins in the tables indicates the non-availability of authentic figures and not the total absence of the vitamin in the foodstuff.

Deficiency of vitamin A

Vitamin A is essential for the healthy functioning of most of the body organs. The effects of deficiency are thus seen in many body tissues. A healthy adult has enough stores of vitamin A in the body to last him for a year or two. Growing children have lesser reserves. Deficiency symptoms appear only after the body stores of the vitamin get depleted and the consequences could be severe.

Night blindness

Night blindness is one of the first detectable signs of vitamin A deficiency. The affected person loses the ability to see in dim light. In the absence of enough vitamin A (retinol), sufficient rhodopsin cannot be regenerated for vision in dim light.

Xerophthalmia

Vitamin A deficiency develops in stages; night blindness progresses to total blindness. The term xerophthalmia means dryness of the eye. The conjunctiva becomes dry and dull. This stage is referred to as conjunctival xerosis. Dry, lusterless patches may be seen on the conjunctiva, and triangular, whitish, foamy spots (Bitot's spots) occur. This is followed by xerosis of the cornea, which becomes dry and hard; a condition called corneal xerosis. Upto this stage, the condition is reversible if a person is properly treated. Dryness can quickly progress to softening of the cornea, known as keratomalacia, which leads to irreversible blindness.

Keratinisation

Due to the absence of vitamin A, the secretions of the mucus are reduced and the epithelial cells become dry and flat. They gradually harden to form keratin (a protein) in a process called keratinisation. When the body is deficient in vitamin A, a number of epithelial tissues undergo keratinisation. With such less mucus, normal digestion and absorption of nutrients falter, worsening the deficiency condition. Similar changes in the cells of other epithelial tissues weaken defenses, causing infections of the respiratory tract, the gastrointestinal tract, the urinary tract, the vagina, and the inner ear. The skin on the body's outer surface also becomes dry and scaly. Small, hard, pigmented lumps of keratin develop at each hair follicle – a condition called follicular hyperkeratosis.

Vitamin A toxicity

Since the human liver has a great storage capacity for vitamin A and some people take mega doses (doses 10 or more times larger than the RDA) of vitamins, there is a possibility of toxic effects. The common symptoms of toxicity (known as hypervitaminosis A) are dry, rough and thick skin, anorexia (loss of appetite), hyperirritability, loss of hair, bone and joint pain, thickening of long bones, bone fragility, headache, enlargement of liver and spleen and hypercalcemia (elevated serum calcium). Vitamin A toxicity in pregnant women results in birth defects. Pregnant women should restrain from taking vitamin A supplements, especially during the first trimester.

Vitamin D

Vitamin D was first recognised by McCollum as the component of 'good fats' that cured rickets. Chemically, compounds with vitamin D activity are sterols. The two forms of the vitamin, which are important, are vitamin D_2 (ergocalciferol) of plant origin and vitamin D_3 (cholecalciferol) of animal origin. Vitamin D_2 is formed when ergosterol (found in plants) is exposed to ultraviolet rays. Vitamin D_3 is the chief form occurring in animal cells and develops in the skin on exposure of 7-dehydrocholesterol to ultraviolet rays from sunshine.

Dietary vitamin D is absorbed along with food fats from the intestine; bile salts are essential for effective absorption. Disease conditions in which fat absorption is affected also hinder vitamin D absorption. Vitamin D made in the skin enters the blood where it circulates attached to a specific protein.

Vitamin D itself is an inactive, storage form of the vitamin concentrated in the liver. It is rapidly hydroxylated (addition of -OH group) to 25-hydroxy vitamin D_3 (calcidiol) in the liver. Calcidiol is further hydroxylated to 1, 25-dihydroxy vitamin D_3 (calcitriol) in the kidney. Calcitriol is considered the active form of the vitamin, which acts as a hormone in calcium metabolism. As vitamin D is necessary for proper bone calcification, it is also called calciferol (to signify an alcohol promoting calcification).

Vitamin D is soluble in fats and organic solvents but insoluble in water. It is stable to heat and is not easily oxidised.

Functions of vitamin D

Vitamin D plays an essential role in the metabolism of calcium and phosphorus. Calcium is required for the development of bones and teeth. Blood calcium levels have to be very tightly maintained for normal functioning of the nervous system. The prohormone vitamin D, which gives rise to the hormone calcitriol, regulates blood calcium levels within a narrow range.

Vitamin D in bone growth

Vitamin D plays a special role in bone growth by making calcium and phosphorus available in the blood. When the blood calcium level becomes too low – for example, when calcium intake from diet is inadequate – the parathyroid gland secretes parathyroid hormone (PTH). PTH promotes the activation of vitamin D to calcitriol, the active form of the vitamin. Calcitriol restores normal blood calcium in three ways – by facilitating absorption of dietary calcium from the intestine, increasing the mobilisation of calcium from the bone into the blood, and increasing the reabsorption and retention of calcium by the kidneys. These actions increase the levels of calcium and phosphorus in the blood. Normal calcium levels permit deposition of calcium in bones and teeth. It is also important for normal nervous function and muscle contraction.

Vitamin D in other roles

Scientists have discovered other roles for vitamin D. Vitamin D has been found in many other tissues such as the brain, nervous system, pancreas, skin, muscles, reproductive organs, liver, kidneys, hormone secreting glands, etc. Vitamin D may have some important role in these tissues as well.

Daily allowances of vitamin D

ICMR has not established a daily allowance of vitamin D for our Indian population, because plenty of sunlight is already available in a tropical country like ours. It is not known how much of vitamin D is exactly required by our body through diet and sunlight. The vitamin D requirement of children is placed between 200-400 International Units (100 IU = 2.5mg). The requirement is lesser for older age groups. The allowance for older age groups is difficult to establish because of exposure to sunlight. Vitamin D requirements have been suggested for different age groups in Table 2.

Table 2
Recommended intake of vitamin D per day

Group	µg	IU
Infants	10	400
Children and adolescents	10	400
Adults (19-22 years)	7.5	300
Adults (22 years onwards)	5	200
Pregnant and lactating women	+5	+200

The requirement for vitamin D can be obtained in great measure through exposure to adequate sunlight. Only in cases where vitamin D requirement is not met through adequate exposure to sunlight or due to metabolic or genetic reasons, therapeutic supplementation of vitamin D may be necessary.

Rich sources of vitamin D

Only a few foods contain vitamin D naturally. Fortunately, the body can make all the vitamin D within itself with the help of a little sunshine.

Vitamin D in foods

Most foods have negligible amounts of vitamin D. Most of the plant foods are poor sources of vitamin D. Some foods of animal origin like egg yolk, liver, fatty fish, butter and fortified milk, provide variable amounts of the vitamin. Vitamin D content of selected foods is given in table 3.

Table 3
Vitamin D content in certain food items

Foodstuff	Vitamin D (IU per 100g)
Milk	1-4
Egg	50-60
Butter	300-100
Egg, yolk	150-400
Fatty fish	200-1,800
Shark liver oil	1,300-5,000
Cod liver oil	8,000-30,000
Halibut liver oil	20,000-4,00,000

Vitamin D from the sun

Most of the world's population relies on natural exposure to sunlight to maintain adequate vitamin D nutrition. The sun imposes no risk to vitamin D toxicity. For most people, exposing hands, face, and arms on a clear summer day for 10 to 15 minutes, at least 3 times a week, should be sufficient to maintain vitamin D nutrition.

Dark-skinned people require longer sunlight exposure than others, to derive the same amount of vitamin D from sunlight exposure. The ultraviolet rays of the sun, which promote vitamin D synthesis, can be blocked by heavy clouds, smoke, or fog. People who are unable to go outdoors frequently or dark-skinned people who live in cloudy or smoggy cities should consume foods fortified with vitamin D or therapeutic supplements to prevent its deficiency.

Deficiency of vitamin D

Vitamin D deficiency is also common in infants who are solely breast-fed without exposure to sunlight. A deficiency of vitamin D leads to inadequate absorption of calcium and phosphorus from the intestine. The amount of bone mineral deposited is reduced. As a result, the shape, structure and strength of bones are affected. In children, the deficiency condition is called rickets and in adults, it is called osteomalacia. In both conditions, the bones become soft, bend easily and are prone to deformities.

Rickets

In infants and children, prolonged vitamin D deficiency leads to rickets. Deposition of calcium in the bones and teeth is faulty, making the bones so weak that they bend when they have to support the body weight. The most common symptoms include bow legs and flat feet. The rib cage becomes deformed with 'beading' or swelling appearing in the ribs. The affected children are potbellied, lethargic and irritable to touch. Rickets can be treated with vitamin D or calcitriol supplements.

Osteomalacia

Osteomalacia is also called 'adult rickets'. 'Osteomalacia' means 'softening of bones'. It occurs due to lack of vitamin D and calcium. It is common in women who subsist on a meagre cereal diet, consume negligible amount of milk products and have little exposure to sunlight. Although adult bones are no longer growing, there is continuous remodelling of the bones. Calcium is continuously removed and deposited in the bones. In adults with prolonged vitamin D deficiency, bone calcium is continuously lost. As a result of bone softening, there is pain in bones of the legs and lower part of the back and general weakness with difficulty in walking and climbing stairs. The bones become fragile and prone to deformities and fractures.

There is high risk for vitamin D deficiency among breast-fed infants and elderly people with little or no exposure to sun, people living in cloudy and smoggy cities, dark-skinned people, women observing purdah system, patients with fat malabsorption disease and kidney failure.

Vitamin D toxicity

Vitamin D toxicity is also called hypervitaminosis D. Vitamin D toxicity does not result from sun exposure. The liver's storage capacity is smaller for vitamin D than for vitamin A. Toxicity results when people take vitamin D doses of 10,000 to 50,000 IU/day over many years.

Excessive amount of vitamin D results in excessive absorption of calcium from the intestine and the elevation of blood calcium levels. Symptoms of toxicity include loss of appetite, nausea, vomiting, diarrhoea, excessive thirst, weight loss, polyuria (excessive urination), severe itching, muscular weakness and joint pain. Excessive blood calcium deposits in the soft tissues such as kidneys leads to formation of stones. Calcium may deposit in the arteries making them hard. This could be dangerous if it occurs in the arteries of the heart and lungs, leading to death.

Vitamin E

In 1922, Evans and Bishop discovered another fat-soluble factor and named it vitamin E. This factor was found to be essential for reproduction in rats. Although the same functions have not been proven in humans, the vitamin was named *tocopherol* (vitamin E) from the Greek *tokos* meaning 'childbirth', *pherein* meaning 'to bear' and *ol* signifying an alcohol.

Vitamin E comprises a group of compounds known as tocopherols and tocotrienols. These are of different types – alpha, beta, gamma and delta. Of these, alpha-tocopherol is the most active and is also the form which is most abundant in foods.

Being fat-soluble in nature, vitamin E and other fat-soluble vitamins are absorbed along with fat in the presence of bile acids. Small amounts of vitamin E are present in all body tissues, but the bulk is stored in muscle, liver, and adipose tissue.

It is now recognised that vitamin E plays a fundamental role in the normal metabolism of all cells. Its deficiency can affect several organ systems. Its functions are related to several other nutrients. Together with some other nutrients, it plays an important role in the defence mechanisms of the body.

Vitamin E is stable to high temperature and acids but it gets oxidised easily in the presence of oxygen. Thus, it acts as an antioxidant. Vitamin E is soluble in fats and organic solvents but insoluble in water. Normal cooking temperatures are not destructive but freezing, processing and frying result in vitamin E losses.

Functions of vitamin E

Vitamin E is a fat-soluble antioxidant and one of body's prime defenders against oxidation. It protects the lipids and other vulnerable components of the body cells and their membranes from oxidation.

Its function as an antioxidant is particularly important in tissues rich in *polyunsaturated fatty acids* (PUFA) and tissues which are in constant contact with oxygen, like lungs. Vitamin E is particularly effective in preventing the oxidation of PUFA, other lipids, as well as related compounds such as vitamin A. Thus, vitamin E protects the lipids of the membranes from oxidative damage due to highly reactive oxygen species and other free radicals. Vitamin E reduces the harmful free radicals to harmless metabolites. This process is called 'free radical scavenging'.

Vitamin E protects the unsaturated lipids and vitamin A because it can accept oxygen and get oxidised itself, thereby acting as an antioxidant. It thus exerts a sparing action on vitamin A by preventing its oxidation. Vitamin E also protects fats and oils from oxidation and rancidity, thereby acting as a preservative.

Recent researches have shown that vitamin E may play a role in reducing the risk of heart disease by protecting LDL (low density lipoprotein) cholesterol against oxidation. Vitamin E exerts an especially important antioxidant effect in the lungs, where the exposure of the cells to oxygen is maximal. Vitamin E's antioxidant property protects not only the lung tissues but also the red blood cells and white blood cells that pass through the lungs. Vitamin E also protects the lungs against air pollutants.

In its antioxidant function, vitamin E acts synergistically with selenium (a trace element) to protect the cells from the damaging effects of oxygen species and free radicals. In fact, selenium and vitamin E both have a sparing effect on each other, and also reduce the body's requirement for each other.

The antioxidant function of vitamin E and other nutrients protects our body against conditions related to oxidative stress, such as aging, air pollution, arthritis, cancer, cardiovascular diseases, diabetes and infections. A lot of research is being conducted on the role of vitamin E in the above mentioned areas.

False hopes

When vitamin E was discovered in 1922, it was termed as the 'antisterility factor' because of its role in fertility and preventing abortions in rats. However, any of these functions have not yet been proven in humans. It is, therefore, a misnomer to call vitamin E the 'reproduction vitamin'. Till date, it has not been proven that vitamin E can improve sexual potency, prevent baldness, improve athletic performance or increase life-span in humans. Nonetheless, vitamin E's role as an antioxidant in protecting the membranes in our bodies from damage, is extremely important.

Daily allowance of vitamin E

There is a paucity of Indian data on the vitamin E content of foods as well as vitamin E requirement by Indian population. Vitamin E deficiency is not prevalent in our country and ICMR has not yet established a daily allowance of vitamin E for our Indian population. Since the requirement for vitamin E depends on the intake of unsaturated essential fatty acids (linoleic and linolenic acids), the requirement for vitamin E suggested is 0.8mg/g of essential fatty acids.

A person consuming a large amount of PUFA needs more vitamin E. Fortunately, vitamin E and PUFA tend to occur together in the same foods.

The Food and Nutrition Board in the United States has recommended levels of vitamin E intake for various age groups. They have been given in table 4.

Table 4
Recommended intake of vitamin E (mg/day)

Group	Age	Males	Females
Infants	0-6 months	4	4
Infants	7-12 months	5	5
Children	1-3 years	6	6
Children	4-8 years	7	7
Children	9-13 years	11	11
Adolescents	14-18 years	15	15
Adults	19 years and above	15	15
Pregnant women	–	-	15
Lactating women	–	-	19

Rich sources of vitamin E

Vitamin E is widespread in foods. Most of the vitamin E in diet comes from vegetarian food, especially vegetable oils and products made from them. Vegetable oils, which are abundant in PUFA, are also the richest sources of vitamin E. Vegetable oils contain 50-100mg vitamin E per 100g oil. Wheat germ oil is very rich in vitamin E with a content of 260mg/100g oil. Corn and soya bean oil rank second; a tablespoon of either is sufficient to meet the day's requirement for vitamin E.

Many dark green, leafy vegetables contain 0.5-1.5mg of vitamin E per 100g of foodstuff. Most of the foods of animal origin are low in vitamin E contents. Breast milk of humans contains adequate vitamin E for the infant but cow's milk is low in vitamin E.

The chief source in Indian diet is thus vegetable oils and whole grain cereals. Coconut oil is an exception with a much lower vitamin E content. An average Indian diet contains about 20g oil which provides 10mg vitamin E, and 400 g of cereal containing 6-8g of fat would provide another 3-4mg of vitamin E. Therefore, vitamin E content in Indian diet is rather satisfactory. In southern India, coconut oil is used for cooking and their diets could be somewhat low in vitamin E content.

A part of vitamin E in vegetable oils may be lost in refining. Vitamin E is readily destroyed by heat such as in deep frying and by oxidation. Thus, fresh and lightly processed foods should be preferred.

The vitamin E content of selected foods in western diets is given in table 5.

Table 5
Vitamin E content in certain food items

Foodstuff	Vitamin E (a-tocopherol equivalents)
Wheat germ oil, 1 tbsp	26.9
Corn oil, 1 tbsp	2.9
Soybean oil, 1 tbsp	2.6
Olive oil, 1 tbsp	1.7
Almond, 1 ounce	6.7

(Note: 1 a-tocopherol equivalents = 1 mg a-tocopherol)

Deficiency of vitamin E

In human beings, vitamin E deficiency is rare. Deficiency is usually seen in patients suffering from fat malabsorption since vitamin E, like other fat-soluble vitamins, is absorbed along with fats. Such patients have multiple vitamin deficiencies. Vitamin E deficiency is also seen in premature infants since they have poor vitamin E stores in their body.

Vitamin E deficiency does not affect the reproductive function in humans as it does in some animals, especially rats. When adequate vitamin E is not available, the cells are more vulnerable to oxidative attack and damage. The lipid in the membranes of red blood cells gets oxidised and the membranes break open. As a result, the cells break open and their contents are lost. This process is known as erythrocyte haemolysis (erythrocyte refers to red blood cells). The continued loss of red blood cells leads to anaemia known as haemolytic anaemia. This condition is commonly seen in premature infants born with small reserves of vitamin E.

In older children and adults, vitamin E deficiency results in a different set of symptoms usually associated with functions of the nervous system and vision. Symptoms include loss of muscle coordination, poor reflexes, decreased sensation in hands and feet, changes in the retina, and impaired vision and speech.

Vitamin E toxicity

Vitamin E is one of the least toxic vitamins. Both humans and animals can safely consume relatively high doses without incurring any side effects. Human beings can tolerate doses, which are 100 times the nutritional requirement. At very high doses, vitamin E can interfere with the utilisation of other fat-soluble vitamins, especially vitamin K. The fat-soluble vitamin K plays an important role in blood clotting. An imbalance in the ratio of vitamin E and vitamin

K can interfere with blood clotting, eventually leading to haemorrhage.

The best recommendation is to use polyunsaturated oils that are rich in vitamin E along with a well-balanced diet without use of mega doses or supplements. Vitamin E may have a role in preventing degenerative disorders such as cardiovascular disorders and cancer. These claims are not fully proven. Therapeutic supplements of vitamin E should be used for patients suffering from fat malabsorption.

Vitamin K

Vitamin K is a fat-soluble vitamin essential for the clotting of blood. If blood does not clot, a single pinprick can drain the entire body of all its blood. Vitamin K acts primarily in blood clotting, where its presence can make the difference between life and death. The 'K' is derived from the Danish word *'koagulation'* meaning blood clotting.

Vitamin K was discovered by Dr. Dam in 1935 as a factor that prevented severe haemorrhage in animals. The factor was named *'koagulationsvitamin'* and subsequently 'vitamin K'. The vitamin was first isolated from alfalfa and Dr. Dam was awarded the Nobel Prize for his discovery.

Several forms of vitamin K have been identified, all of them belonging to a group of chemical compounds called *quinones*. Phylloquinone (vitamin K_1) is the major form found in plant foods and was initially isolated from alfalfa by Dr. Dam. It is our dietary form of vitamin K. Menaquinone (vitamin K_2) is synthesised by the bacteria in our intestinal tract. Vitamin K_1 and K_2 are natural, fat-soluble forms of the vitamin. Menadione (vitamin K_3) is a synthetic, water-soluble form of the vitamin, which is two to three times more potent than the natural vitamin. Being water-soluble, vitamin K_3 does not require the presence of bile for absorption.

Like other fat-soluble vitamins, vitamin K is absorbed along with fat in the presence of bile acids. Our body does not maintain large stores of vitamin K unlike other fat-soluble vitamins. Vitamin K is rapidly cleared from the body in urine. However, the small amount of vitamin K in the body is recycled and used again.

Vitamin K is fat-soluble, resistant to heat, but easily destroyed by acids, light and oxidising agents.

Functions of vitamin K

Vitamin K has an important function in the clotting of blood. Several steps in the blood-clotting process depend on vitamin K. Recent research has also explored some role of vitamin K in bone development.

Role of vitamin K in blood clotting

Normally, blood flows in our body without clotting. But when bleeding occurs because of injury, the blood clots and the bleeding is stopped. The clot is made of fibrin, a protein that gets deposited in the form of fine threads to form a network. The formation of fibrin is not a one-step process but a series of events, which requires a number of clotting factors. These clotting factors are proteins, which are synthesised by liver in an inactive form. The activation of four of these factors, including factors II, VII, IX and X, requires vitamin K. The activated factors can bind with calcium (which is also essential in blood clotting) and then participate in the blood clotting process. Vitamin K is thus essential for the clotting of blood.

Role of vitamin K in bone development

Vitamin K also participates in the synthesis of bone proteins. Osteocalcin is a protein present in the bone, which binds calcium and is involved in bone development. This protein is dependent on vitamin K; without vitamin K, it cannot bind calcium.

Daily allowances of vitamin K

It has been difficult to determine an allowance for dietary vitamin K intake, partly because it is synthesised in our intestines in variable amounts and partly because of the paucity of data on vitamin K requirements and contents in foods.

ICMR has not established RDA for vitamin K for our Indian population.

The Food and Nutrition Board in the United States has established a range of 'estimated safe and adequate daily dietary intakes' of vitamin K. The vitamin is produced by our intestinal bacteria in variable amounts, and our body has small reserves of the vitamin. The Board has recommended an intake of 1-2mg of vitamin K per kg body weight. The lower amount is based on the assumption that about half of the requirement is met by bacterial synthesis. The upper value is calculated assuming that the entire requirement is supplied by the diet.

Vitamin K requirements for different age groups is given in table 6.

Table 6
Recommended intake of vitamin K (mg /day)

Group	Age	Males	Females
Infants	0-6 months	5	5
Infants	7-12 months	10	10
Children	1-3 years	15	15
Children	4-6 years	20	20
Children	7-10 years	30	30
Children	11-14 years	45	45
Adolescents	15-18 years	65	55
Adults	19-24 years	70	60
Adults	25 years and above	80	65
Pregnant women	-	-	65
Lactating women	-	-	65

Older adults who have chronic diseases, are on drug therapy, or are consuming poor diets may need higher amounts. Newborns, especially premature babies, require a vitamin K injection shortly after birth.

Rich sources of vitamin K

Vitamin K is found in large amounts in green leafy vegetables, especially broccoli, spinach, kale, cabbage, turnip greens, and dark lettuce, usually at levels greater than 100mg/100g. A single serving of the leafy vegetables can usually provide more than the day's allowance. The amount of vitamin in dairy products, meats and eggs tend to be variable, 1-50mg/100g and fruits and cereals usually contain about 15mg/100g.

The average vitamin K content of selected foods in western diets is given in table 7.

Breast milk tends to be low in vitamin K content, providing insufficient amount of vitamin for infants less than 6 months.

Vitamin K is fairly stable. It is not destroyed by ordinary cooking methods nor is it lost in cooking water. It is however, sensitive to light.

Table 7
Vitamin K content in certain food items

Foodstuff	Vitamin K (mg)
Spinach, ½ cup	131
Broccoli, ½ cup	63
Cabbage, ½ cup	52
Lettuce, 1 leaf	22
Turnip greens, ½ cup (cooked)	82
Tomato, 1	28
Chick-pea, 1 ounce	74
Whole wheat flour, 1 cup	36
Soybean oil, 1 tablespoon	76
Milk (cow), 1 ounce	1.25
Milk (human), 1 ounce	0.6
Pork, 3.5 ounce	88
Egg, 1 large	25

Deficiency of vitamin K

Primary vitamin K deficiency (deficiency due to inadequate intake) is rare. Even though our body stores a limited amount of vitamin K, a shortage of vitamin K is unlikely, since it is derived from both food and bacterial synthesis in our intestine. Green leafy vegetables are high in vitamin K, fruits and cereals are low, and meat and dairy products are intermediate in vitamin K content.

Excess of vitamin K deficiency results in impaired blood clotting; symptoms include easy bruising, nosebleeds, bleeding gums, blood in the urine and stools, or extremely heavy menstrual bleeding. Deficiency in infants may result in life-threatening bleeding, leading to haemorrhage.

Vitamin K deficiency may occur when the absorption of fat and related substances is abnormal, due to long-term antibiotic therapy which results in sterilisation of the gut, when anticoagulant drugs have been used to prevent blood clotting, immediately after birth because bacteria are not present in the gastrointestinal tract, and severe liver disease.

Deficiency due to fat malabsorption

Being fat-soluble, vitamin K requires the presence of bile acids for absorption. Any condition affecting the flow of bile, resulting in fat malabsorption also affects the absorption of vitamin K. Absorption of vitamin K is affected due to diarrhoea, obstruction of the biliary tract and severe liver damage affecting bile synthesis. When absorption is inadequate, supplements of vitamin K should be given along with bile salts to promote absorption.

Deficiency due to antibiotic therapy

Antibiotic therapy sterilises the intestinal tract, killing all the bacteria present. Intestinal bacteria contribute significantly to our daily vitamin K needs. Long-term antibiotic therapy along with a poor diet can lead to vitamin K deficiency and should be accompanied by good supplements of vitamin K.

Deficiency due to anticoagulant therapy

Anticoagulant drugs and blood thinners are often used in the treatment of certain heart diseases such as coronary thrombosis. The action of these drugs is antagonistic to vitamin K and they prevent the formation of blood clotting factor II. Anticoagulant therapy carries the risk of haemorrhage. When an excessive amount of anticoagulant is given, vitamin K supplements should be given to counteract it.

Heamorrhagic disease in newborns

Newborns may develop heamorrhagic diseases due to lack of vitamin K because:
- The intestinal tract is sterile and intestinal bacteria have not yet established themselves
- Breast milk contains only 20% of the RDA for an infant
- Blood clotting factors are not fully developed
- Vitamin K regeneration cycle is not fully developed

Premature infants are more susceptible to vitamin K deficiency because of poor transfer of vitamin K through the placenta. Newborns are often given a single injection of vitamin K after birth to prevent deficiency.

Large amounts of vitamin A and E also interfere with the absorption and metabolism of vitamin K.

Vitamin K toxicity

There is no known toxicity associated with high doses of phylloquinone (vitamin K_1), a natural form of vitamin K. However, when menadione (vitamin K_3), a synthetic form, is given in large doses, especially to infants and pregnant women, toxicity can occur. High doses of vitamin K can also reduce the effectiveness of anticoagulant drugs. Toxicity symptoms include jaundice, red blood cell haemolysis and brain damage.

Water-soluble Vitamins

B complex vitamins (including thiamin, riboflavin, niacin, vitamin B_6, pantothenic acid, biotin, folic acid, vitamin B_{12}), and vitamin C are usually referred to as water-soluble vitamins. However, their solubility in water is the only characteristic that they share. Because of this general characteristic, these vitamins are easily absorbed by simple diffusion and do not require the presence of fat or bile acids for their absorption.

The discoveries of the water-soluble vitamins began at the turn of the last century with the recognition by Christian Eijkman, a Dutch physician, that rice bran contained a factor that prevented beriberi in certain animals. The factor was called water-soluble B factor. Another water-soluble factor, which prevented scurvy, was discovered later, and named vitamin C. By this time, it was clear that water-soluble B was not a single factor but a group of biologically active factors with similar physical properties and food sources. Collectively, these factors became known as the 'B complex'.

Water-soluble vitamins have their own unique set of characteristics. Each of the B vitamins contains nitrogen, which is lacking in vitamin C and other fat-soluble vitamins. Most of the water-soluble vitamins function as essential coenzymes or cofactors of enzymes* involved in various aspects of metabolism. A cofactor or coenzyme is a small molecule that associates closely with enzymes and facilitates their functioning. As vital coenzymes, vitamin B is required for normal growth, nerve and brain function, reproduction and almost every cellular reaction in the body.

It is true that without B vitamins, the body would lack energy. However, vitamins do not provide the body with fuel for energy. The energy yielding nutrients are carbohydrates, fats and proteins. B vitamins help the body to use that fuel. Several of the B vitamins – thiamin, riboflavin, niacin, pantothenic acid and biotin – form part of the coenzymes that enable enzymes to release energy from carbohydrates, fats, and proteins. Other B vitamins also play indispensable roles in metabolism. Vitamin B_6 assists enzymes that

---

* Enzymes are proteins that catalyse or speed up metabolic reactions in the body.

metabolise amino acids (basic unit of proteins), and folic acid, and B_{12} help cells to multiply.

Since the water-soluble vitamins are not stored in the body for more than a few days, daily or frequent consumption is imperative. On the same account, they rarely accumulate in amounts that can cause toxicity. Since the water-soluble vitamins simultaneously exist in the food sources, rarely will your body be deficient of only one of the B vitamins; usually the deficiency is of two or three of them.

Thiamin

Thiamin or vitamin B_1 was one of the first B vitamins to be discovered and elucidated. The discovery of thiamin provided the answer to the puzzle of beriberi. Beriberi is a disease associated with the consumption of highly polished rice. It was widely prevalent in Asia, and had plagued Asian population for centuries. In 1890, Christian Eijkman, a Dutch physician noticed polyneuritis (a symptom of beriberi) in chicken that were fed polished rice. The symptoms disappeared when the diet was changed to whole grain brown rice. In 1936, Dr. R R Williams identified the structure of thiamin. The vitamin was called thiamin from *thio* (sulfur containing) and *amine* (nitrogen).

Since thiamin is water-soluble, it is actively transported across the small intestine. This process is, however, inhibited by alcohol consumption. Chronic alcohol consumption is associated with thiamin deficiency.

Thiamin is distributed throughout the body but it is not stored in significant amounts in any organ. Highest concentrations are found in the heart, brain, liver and kidney. Thiamin is stable to heat in the dry form. However, it is readily destroyed by cooking.

Functions of thiamin

The principal functioning form of thiamin is Thiamin Pyrophosphate (TPP). Conversion of thiamin to TPP involves phosphorylation (addition of phosphorus) and requires a molecule of energy called adenosine triphosphate (ATP). TPP acts as a coenzyme in several important metabolic reactions – oxidative decarboxylation and transketolation reactions.

Thiamin functions in the metabolism of carbohydrates, fats and proteins. The carbohydrate in our diet is digested to form glucose – the simplest carbohydrate and the chief fuel for our body. Glucose is converted to a series of compounds in the body, resulting in slow oxidation in stages. Pyruvic acid is an important compound in this series and this compound requires thiamin in the form of TPP for its further metabolism. In thiamin deficiency, pyruvic acid fails to get oxidised and gets converted to lactic acid, which accumulates in the tissues. Since glucose is the main fuel for the body and the only fuel used by the brain, the consequences of its deficiency can be serious.

TPP is required at another point in carbohydrate metabolism. It is required for the metabolism of another compound called alpha-ketoglutaric acid. This compound is also obtained from fats and proteins; hence thiamin is essential for the metabolism of all three energy-giving nutrients – carbohydrates, fats and proteins.

TPP has also been found to be concentrated in nerve and muscle cells. Thiamin may be involved in some aspects of the function of nerve cell membranes and may influence the functioning of neurotransmitters as well.

Daily allowances of thiamin

Thiamin requirements are closely related to carbohydrate and energy intake and hence, its requirement is usually expressed in terms of milligrams per 1000 cal of energy intake. ICMR has established an RDA of 0.5 mg per 1000 cal consumed.

Ordinary diet consumed by the poor people in our country is heavily based on cereals and not much of pulses which provide about 0.8mg thiamin per 1000 cal, and those based on polished rice provide 0.3mg per 1000 cal. However, upper class diet based on polished rice provides larger amounts of thiamin because of the greater consumption of foods such as pulses, vegetables and milk.

Daily thiamin requirement varies between 0.5–2mg/day depending upon age, physiological status and level of physical activity. Thiamin requirement for Indian population of different age groups is given in table 8.

Table 8
Recommended intake of thiamin (mg/day)

Group	Age	Males	Females
Infants	0-6 months	55ug/kg	55ug/kg
Infants	7-12 months	50ug/kg	50ug/kg
Children	1-3 years	0.6ug/kg	0.6ug/kg
Children	4-6 years	0.9ug/kg	0.9ug/kg
Children	7-9 years	1.0ug/kg	1.0ug/kg
Children	10-12 years	1.1ug/kg	1.0ug/kg
Adolescents	13-15 years	1.2ug/kg	1.0ug/kg
Adolescents	16-18 years	1.3ug/kg	1.0ug/kg
Adults	Sedentary work	1.2ug/kg	0.9ug/kg
Adults	Moderate work	1.4ug/kg	1.1ug/kg
Adults	Heavy work	1.6ug/kg	1.2ug/kg
Pregnant	-	-	+0.2ug/kg
Lactating women	0-6 months	-	+0.3ug/kg
Lactating women	6-12 months	-	+0.2ug/kg

Rich sources of thiamin

It is widely distributed in many foods. The richest sources include yeast, wheat germ and liver, but these do not form an important part of most diets. The cereal grains comprise the most important source of thiamin in our diets. Whole grain cereals and legumes contribute significantly to our daily thiamin intake. However, most of the thiamin in the grains is found in the outer layer, much of which is removed during milling. Highly polished rice and refined flour are therefore poor sources. Parboiled rice is a much better source as the outer layer is intact during parboiling. Fermented products such as 'idli' are much better sources since thiamin content increases during fermentation.

Animal foods including milk are relatively poor sources of thiamin. Egg is a fair source of thiamin, most of which is concentrated in the yolk. Peas, soyabeans and peanuts are excellent sources of thiamin.

Although the concentration of thiamin in vegetables and fruits is low, the intake should be such that they make important contribution to the daily diet. Milk is likewise a fair source if taken daily in good amounts. An exhaustive list of thiamin content of all commonly consumed foods is given in Appendix II.

Thiamin can be easily destroyed by heat, oxidation and radiation, but it is stable during freezing. Cooking losses of thiamin tend to be variable depending upon cooking time, method, temperature, pH, quantity of water used, etc.

Uncooked fish, shrimps and clams contain thiaminase, an enzyme that destroys thiamin. Usually, this enzyme presents no problem since it is easily destroyed by cooking. Tea and a few other foods contain certain compounds that act as thiamin antagonists. Such foods should be consumed only in moderation.

Deficiency of thiamin

Since thiamin is required for the metabolism of carbohydrates, fats and proteins, a wide range of symptoms develop due to deficiency. The deficiency condition is called beriberi, which literally means 'I cannot'. The clinical effects of deficiency are reflected in the gastrointestinal system, the nervous system, the cardiovascular system, and the musculoskeletal system.

Gastrointestinal system

Various symptoms such as anorexia (loss of appetite), indigestion and constipation may occur. When the cells of the secretory glands of the gastrointestinal system, GI, tract do not receive sufficient energy from glucose, they cannot do their work in digestion to produce more glucose. A vicious cycle of deficiency ensues, leading to weight loss.

Nervous system

The central nervous system is extremely dependent on glucose as fuel, especially the brain, which uses glucose almost exclusively as its source of fuel. Deficiency of thiamin results in reduced alertness, impaired reflex actions, general apathy, and lack of interest and fatigue. This condition is often referred to as 'dry beriberi'. There is increasing nerve irritation, pain, numbness and burning sensation in feet and cramping of calf muscles. Severe deficiency may ultimately progress to paralysis.

Cardiovascular system

With continuing thiamin deficiency, the heart muscle weakens, resulting in cardiac failure. As a result of cardiac failure, oedema appears in the lower limbs followed by the thighs. The characteristic swelling in the legs due to oedema is referred to as 'wet beriberi'. The patient experiences difficulty in breathing and the heart gets enlarged. Even death may occur due to cardiac impairments.

Wernicke-Korsakoff syndrome

It is a neurological disorder resulting from thiamin deficiency in chronic alcoholics. The symptoms include abnormal eye movements, staggering gait (walk), and abnormalities in mental function ranging from confusion and amnesia to coma.

Riboflavin

Riboflavin is a water-soluble B-complex vitamin also known as vitamin B_2. It was first recognised as a yellow-green fluorescent pigment in milk in 1879. The vitamin was synthesised and named riboflavin in 1935. Riboflavin gets its name from its colour and its component sugar, ribose. Pigments that have fluorescent properties are designated as 'flavins'. Later it was found that the yellow-green fluorescent compound had a sugar 'ribose' attached to it, and hence the name riboflavin.

Riboflavin is absorbed from the small intestine, where it is phosphorylated (addition of phosphorus). It is not stored in our body in significant amounts, therefore, it must be supplied in the diet regularly. Small amounts of the vitamin are stored in the liver, kidney and heart.

Riboflavin is an orange-yellow crystalline substance, insoluble in fats and dissolves sparingly in water to give a characteristic greenish-yellow fluorescence. Riboflavin is stable to heat, oxidation and acids; however, it is easily destroyed by visible light and the ultraviolet rays of the sun.

Functions of riboflavin

Riboflavin is essential for the metabolism of carbohydrates, amino acids and lipids and also supports antioxidant protective function. It discharges these functions in the form of two coenzymes, riboflavin monophosphate or Flavin Mononucleotide (FMN) and Flavin Adenine Dinucleotide (FAD). The conversion of riboflavin into its coenzyme forms requires energy in the form of ATP molecules. Riboflavin is first converted to FMN; most FMN is converted to FAD.

The flavin coenzymes FMN and FAD are versatile coenzymes that participate in a number of oxidation-reduction reactions. Both these coenzymes act as hydrogen acceptors. A series of reactions takes place in the energy cycle (TCA cycle or Kreb's cycle) by which ATP is generated. Each step is catalysed by enzymes and the process involves transfer of hydrogen from one compound to another until eventually it reaches oxygen and forms water. FMN and FAD act as coenzymes for the enzymes that catalyse these reactions.

FMN and FAD are also coenzymes for dehydrogenase enzymes that catalyse the oxidation of fatty acids. FMN is also required for the conversion of vitamin B_6 (pyridoxine) to its active form. FAD is also required for the synthesis of the B-complex vitamin niacin from the amino acid tryptophan in our body.

Another enzyme called glutathione reductase requires FAD as coenzyme. This enzyme plays a major role in protecting organisms from reactive oxygen species that can cause oxidative damage to body tissues. Together with niacin-containing coenzymes, riboflavin helps to combat oxidative damage to the cell.

Daily allowances of riboflavin

Riboflavin requirements are related to the total energy needs, body size, metabolic rate, rate of growth, and the actual energy intake. Riboflavin requirements are also expressed in terms of milligrams per 1000 cal of energy intake. ICMR has established an RDA of 0.6mg per 1000 cal consumed after allowing for cooking losses.

The daily safe requirement of this vitamin ranges from 0.7 to 2.2mg/day depending upon age, physiological status and level of activity. Riboflavin requirement for Indians of different age groups is given in table 9.

Table 9
Recommended intake of riboflavin (mg/day)

Group	Age	Males	Females
Infants	0-6 months	55 µg/kg	55 µg/kg
Infants	7-12 months	50 µg/kg	50 µg/kg
Children	1-3 years	0.6 µg/kg	0.6 µg/kg
Children	4-6 years	0.9 µg/kg	0.9 µg/kg
Children	7-9 years	1.0 µg/kg	1.0 µg/kg
Children	10-12 years	1.1 µg/kg	1.0 µg/kg
Adolescents	13-15 years	1.2 µg/kg	1.0 µg/kg
Adolescents	16-18 years	1.3 µg/kg	1.0 µg/kg
Adults	Sedentary work	1.2 µg/kg	0.9 µg/kg
Adults	Moderate work	1.4 µg/kg	1.1 µg/kg
Adults	Heavy work	1.6 µg/kg	1.2 µg/kg
Pregnant women	0-6 months	-	+0.2 µg/kg
Lactating women	-	-	+0.3 µg/kg

Riboflavin requirements increase in certain conditions such as fever, stress of injury, surgery, malabsorption disorders, increase in physical activity, growth period such as childhood, pregnancy and lactation, and hyperthyroidism.

Poor Indian diets provide 0.3-0.6 mg/1000 cal. However, if milk is consumed in adequate amounts, the day's riboflavin requirement can be easily met.

Rich sources of riboflavin

Riboflavin is widely distributed in foods. Animal foods are by far, the best sources of riboflavin. Milk, milk products such as cheese, and liver are the richest sources of riboflavin. No other commonly eaten food than milk and milk products can make such a substantial contribution in a single serving.

Among plant foods, leafy vegetables are good sources. In diets based on vegetarian foods, riboflavin tends to be a limiting nutrient but the content of such diets can be increased by a more liberal intake of greens and frequent use of sprouted and fermented foods. Riboflavin content of food increases during germination and fermentation.

Meat, egg and cereals are also fair sources of riboflavin. However, milling and refining result in large losses of the vitamin. Flours are generally low in riboflavin unless they are enriched, as is commonly practised in western countries. Fruits, roots and tubers are poor sources of riboflavin, and fats and oils are practically devoid of the vitamin. Riboflavin content of commonly consumed foods is given in Appendix II.

Ultraviolet light and radiation destroy riboflavin. For this reason, milk should not be sold in clear glass bottles or transparent plastic packages.

Deficiency of riboflavin

Ariboflavinosis is the medical name for clinical riboflavin deficiency. Riboflavin deficiency is rarely found in isolation; it frequently occurs in combination with deficiencies of other water-soluble vitamins. Deficiency of riboflavin is common in our country because of the lack of animal foods rich in the vitamin.

A deficiency of riboflavin results in clinical symptoms such as changes in lips, tongue, corners of the lips and eyes. The early symptoms include photophobia, burning and itching of the eyes, soreness and burning of lips, mouth and tongue. The lips become dry and chaffed, a condition called cheilosis; the tongue becomes red and shiny (glossitis) and develops fissures with yellowish color (fissured tongue). The angles at the corners of the mouth become ulcerated (angular stomatitis). Skin becomes scaly and greasy around the skin folds (seborrhoeic dermatitis).

The conjunctiva becomes red and inflamed, and eyelids appear swollen and become sticky. They also become abnormally sensitive to light and get easily fatigued. Blurring of vision, itching, watering and soreness of the eye may occur as well. Extra blood vessels develop in the cornea of the eye and it looks red and bloody (corneal vascularisation).

Deficiency in newborns

Newborn infants suffering from jaundice are often given phototherapy. Since riboflavin is light sensitive, such infants may develop riboflavin deficiency unless sufficient supplements are provided.

Niacin

Niacin deficiency disease *pellagra* was first identified in 1735 by Casals. After extensive research, Goldberger held in 1918 that the cause of the disease was due to nutrient deficiency. However, it was in 1937 that Elvehjem ascertained that pellagra was caused due to deficiency of a water-soluble B vitamin, called niacin.

Niacin is the generic term for two compounds, nicotinic acid and nicotinamide. Both have equal biologic activity and potency. It was also established early that the amino acid tryptophan gets converted to niacin in our body. Thus, a diet liberal in protein would provide enough niacin even though the diet may be low in niacin. In the body, 60mg of tryptophan yields 1mg niacin. Since the body obtains niacin both from diet and from the amino acid tryptophan, niacin value is expressed in terms of niacin equivalents (NE).

1NE=1mg niacin=60mg tryptophan

Being water-soluble, niacin is directly absorbed from the small intestine. The body does not have large reserves of the vitamin and it should be supplied regularly in the diet. Any excess of the vitamin is excreted in the urine.

Niacin is moderately soluble in hot water. It is very stable to heat, light, oxidation, acids and alkalis. Even boiling and autoclaving does not destroy it.

Functions of niacin

Like other B-complex vitamins, niacin is a constituent of coenzymes involved in important metabolic pathways such as oxidation of glucose, fat synthesis and in tissue respiration. However, niacin is also used as a drug in treatment of some disorders.

Niacin as a constituent of coenzymes

Niacin is a partner with riboflavin in the cellular coenzyme systems. In these systems the oxidation of glucose often takes place in the absence of oxygen simply by the removal of hydrogen ions. These ions are passed down the line from one compound to another to the eventual receiver oxygen, forming water and carbon dioxide. The two niacin coenzymes that operate in these metabolic reactions are NAD (nicotinamide adenine dinucleotide) and NADP (nicotinamide adenine dinucleotide phosphate). NAD and NADP act as coenzymes for more than 200 enzymes involved in the metabolism of carbohydrates, fatty acids and amino acids.

NAD and NADP are hydrogen acceptors involved in a large number of oxidation-reduction reactions. On accepting hydrogen, they become NADH and NADPH respectively. In general, NAD is involved in catabolic reactions and NADP in anabolic (synthetic) reactions.

Niacin as a drug

Pharmacologic doses of niacin are used in cardiovascular diseases to lower elevated serum cholesterol and triglycerides. However, niacin should be used with caution as a drug because it can produce side effects such as skin flushing, itching, tingling sensation and gastrointestinal disturbances.

Daily allowances of niacin

Niacin requirements depend on a number of factors such as age, body size, level of physical activity, growth periods, and physiological conditions such as pregnancy, lactation and illness.

Since niacin takes part in a number of reactions of energy metabolism, its requirement also has been related to energy requirement. The ICMR has recommended an intake of 6.6mg NE per 1000 cal. The daily requirement of niacin varies from 8-26mg NE for various age groups. Niacin requirement for Indian population of different age groups is given in table 10.

Table 10
Recommended intake of niacin (mg NE/day)

Group	Age	Males	Females
Infants	0-6 months	710 µg/kg	710 µg/kg
Infants	7-12 months	650 µg/kg	650 µg/kg
Children	1-3 years	8µg/kg	8µg/kg
Children	4-6 years	11µg/kg	11µg/kg
Children	7-9 years	13µg/kg	13µg/kg
Children	10-12 years	15µg/kg	15µg/kg
Adolescents	13-15 years	16µg/kg	14µg/kg
Adolescents	16-18 years	17µg/kg	14µg/kg
Adults	Sedentary work	16µg/kg	12µg/kg
Adults	Moderate work	18µg/kg	14µg/kg
Adults	Heavy work	21µg/kg	16µg/kg
Pregnant women	-	-	+2µg/kg
Lactating women	0-6 months	-	+4µg/kg
Lactating women	6-12 months	-	+3µg/kg

As with the other B-complex vitamins, the niacin requirements are increased whenever metabolism is increased as in fevers, injury or surgery.

Rich sources of niacin

Normally, a diet that provides adequate amount of protein would also provide enough niacin since tryptophan is converted to niacin, and most of the protein rich foods (except for milk) are also good sources of niacin. Milk and egg contain small amounts of niacin, but they are excellent sources of tryptophan, giving them good NE (Niacin Equivalents) contents. A diet containing both plant and animal foods and containing adequate protein provides about 10-11mg NE from tryptophan, which is more than half the RDA for a normal adult.

Organ meats like liver and kidney, peanuts and yeast are rich sources of niacin, but they do not form a significant part of our diet. Meat, fish and chicken are also rich in niacin.

Whole cereals and grains are fair sources of niacin. However, niacin in whole grains is bound to some carbohydrates to form complexes called niacytin. The niacin bound in this complex is not released after digestion and is unavailable to the body. Treatment of cereals with alkali, such as lime, releases much of the bound niacin. The American tradition of soaking maize in lime before making corn tortillas increases the amount of available niacin.

In our country, diets based on maize and jowar provide about 5.0mg NE per 1000 cal, whereas those based on milled rice, parboiled rice and mixed grains provide 6.0, 12.0 and 10.0mg NE per 1000 cal taking into account the tryptophan content of the diet.

Potatoes, legumes and some green leafy vegetables provide fair amounts of niacin, but most fruits and vegetables are poor sources. Niacin content of commonly consumed foods is given in Appendix II. Values given in tables give only the niacin content of food stuffs; they do not take into account the contribution of tryptophan to the total NE of the diet, and hence they are an underestimate of the niacin value of the foods.

Cooking of foods does not result in any significant losses of niacin nor does it significantly increase availability of the bound niacin in whole grains. Sprouting and fermentation are associated with 50% increase in niacin content.

Deficiency of niacin

The first symptoms of niacin deficiency are general, such as weakness, anorexia (loss of appetite), laziness, indigestion and various skin eruptions.

Severe deficiency of niacin leads to pellagra, which is characterised by the 3 D's, dermatitis, diarrhoea and dementia and sometimes the fourth D, death.

The dermatologic symptoms are the most prominent. The skin develops dark, pigmented, scaly dermatitis in sun-exposed areas. There is a characteristic symmetric dermatitis, especially on the exposed parts of the body – hands, forearms, elbows, feet, legs, knees and neck. The skin first becomes red, swollen and tender. If untreated, it turns rough, cracked and scaly. The word 'pellagra' comes from the Italian word for 'rough skin'.

Digestive abnormalities cause irritation and inflammation of the mucous membranes of the mouth and gastrointestinal tract. There is soreness in tongue, mouth and throat, with glossitis extending throughout the gastrointestinal tract. The patient may also experience nausea, vomiting, diarrhoea and abdominal pain.

Some patients also experience neurological symptoms such as depression, apathy, fatigue, confusion, dizziness, dementia, poor memory, irritability and hallucinations.

Niacin toxicity

Our body has small reserves of niacin and it rarely builds up in toxic amounts. However, pharmacologic doses of niacin used in treatment of cardiovascular disorders can produce symptoms such as flushing. Niacin administered in large doses dilates the capillaries and causes a painful, tingling sensation, and causes flushing. Large doses of niacin used to lower blood cholesterol can also cause adverse side effects such as liver damage and peptic ulcers. Megadoses of vitamins should be monitored carefully because high doses are medication and not nutritional supplements.

Vitamin B_6

Vitamin B_6 is a water-soluble B-complex vitamin that was first isolated in the 1930s. In 1934, Gyorgy reported that vitamin B_2 consists of two factors – riboflavin and vitamin B_6 that prevented skin lesions in rats. Vitamin B_6 was isolated in 1938 by several laboratories and its chemical structure was identified soon after.

There are six forms of vitamin B_6 – pyridoxine, pyridoxal, pyridoxamine and their phosphate derivatives, pyridoxine phosphate, pyridoxal phosphate and pyridoxamine phosphate. In the body, all the three forms are equally active as precursors of the coenzyme form of the vitamin.

Since vitamin B_6 is water-soluble, it is easily absorbed from the small intestine. The body stores of this vitamin are small, although small amounts are found throughout the body tissues. The greatest levels are found in liver, brain, kidney, spleen and muscle. Muscle serves as the largest depot of the body stores of vitamin B_6.

Vitamin B_6 is water-soluble, heat-stable and acid-stable. However, it is sensitive to light and alkalis. Of the various forms, pyridoxine is more resistant to food processing and storage conditions, and probably represents the principle form in food products.

Functions of vitamin B_6

The coenzyme form of vitamin B_6 is Pyridoxal Phosphate (PLP). PLP plays a vital role in the functioning of approximately 100 enzymes, most of which are involved in amino acid metabolism. Amino acids are building blocks of proteins, hence vitamin B_6 plays a vital role in protein metabolism, unlike the previous three water-soluble vitamins which are required for metabolism of all three energy yielding nutrients – carbohydrates, fats and proteins. Here are few examples of enzyme systems which depend on vitamin B_6.

Decarboxylation

It involves removal of carboxyl group (COOH). This reaction converts glutamic acid (an amino acid) to GABA (Gamma Amino Butyric Acid, a substance found in the gray matter of the brain. Decarboxylation also converts tryptophan (an amino acid) to serotonin, a neurotransmitter.

Transamination
This reaction involves transfer of amino group ($-NH_2$) from one compound to another forming amino acids. Transamination reactions enable us to synthesise several amino acids within our body even if we do not get them from our diet in sufficient amounts.

Transulphuration
This involves the removal and transfer of sulphur groups from one amino acid to another.

Tryptophan conversion to niacin
In the previous chapter, it was mentioned that niacin can be synthesised from tryptophan in our body. This conversion is a multistep process, one of which is catalysed by vitamin B_6. Thus, adequate vitamin B_6 in the diet reduces the requirement for dietary niacin.

Haemoglobin synthesis
PLP functions as a coenzyme in the synthesis of haeme, a component of haemoglobin. Haemoglobin is found in the red blood cells and its deficiency leads to anaemia.

Nucleic acid synthesis
PLP acts as a coenzyme for a key enzyme involved in the synthesis of nucleic acids (DNA and RNA).

Pyridoxal phosphate is also required for deamination reactions, for the breakdown of glycogen to glucose, for formation of antibodies, and probably for the synthesis of unsaturated fatty acids in the body.

Vitamin B_6 supplements are also used in pharmacologic doses for the treatment of certain conditions such as premenstrual syndrome, depression, and nausea and vomiting during pregnancy.

Daily allowances of vitamin B_6

The need for vitamin B_6 is proportional to the protein intake and the protein metabolised. Vitamin B_6 requirements however are not expressed in terms of protein intake. ICMR has suggested daily allowances of vitamin B_6 for different age groups in our Indian population. A daily intake of 0.6 to 2.5mg of vitamin B_6 would meet the requirement of different age groups. Requirement increases during periods such as pregnancy and lactation when protein requirements also increase. The daily allowances for different age groups is shown in table 11.

Table 11
Recommended intake of vitamin B_6 (mg/day)

Group	Age	mg/day
Infants	0-6 months	0.1
Infants	7-12 months	0.4
Children	1-3 years	0.9
Children	4-6 years	0.9
Children	7-9 years	1.6
Children	10-12 years	1.6
Adolescents	13-15 years	2.0
Adolescents	16-18 years	2.0
Adults	18 and above	2.0
Pregnant women	-	2.5
Lactating women	-	2.5

Rich sources of vitamin B_6

Vitamin B_6 is widespread in foods, but many sources provide only small amounts. Whole grains are good sources of vitamin B_6 but most of this is lost in the milling of grains. In addition, the availability of the vitamin in cereals and legumes may be limited because of binding to other components such as plant fibre. In general, bioavailability of vitamin B_6 obtained from animal foods is better than those obtained from plant foods.

Other good sources include liver, kidney, other meats and seeds. Pulses, leafy vegetables, groundnuts and vegetables such as potatoes also contain generous amounts of Vitamin B_6. Among fruits, banana is rich in vitamin B_6. Milk and egg contain limited amounts of the vitamin. Some amount of vitamin B_6 is lost from foods during cooking.

The vitamin B_6 content of Indian foods has not been systematically studied. Table 12 gives the vitamin B_6 content of selected foods in western diets.

Table 12
Vitamin B6 content in certain food items

Foodstuff	Vitamin B_6 (mg)
Bread, whole wheat, 1 slice	0.05
Rice, brown, 1 cup	0.28
Rice, white, 1 cup	0.15
Wheat germ, ¼ cup	0.28
Broccoli, boiled, ½ cup	0.15
Cauliflower, cooked, ½ cup	0.11
Carrot, 1 medium	0.11
Potato, baked, 1 medium	0.70
Spinach, cooked, 1 cup	0.44
Apple, 1 medium	0.07
Banana, 1 medium	0.66

Foodstuff	Vitamin B_6 (mg)
Orange juice, 1 cup	0.10
Beef, liver, 3.5 ounce	0.91
Chicken, 3.5 ounce	0.60
Egg, 1 large	0.07
Peanuts, roasted, 1 ounce	0.07
Walnut, 1 ounce	0.16
Cashew nut, 1 ounce	0.07
Lentil, boiled, 1 cup	0.35
Soyabean, boiled, 1 cup	0.40
Milk, 1 cup	0.10
Milk (human), 1 cup	0.03

Deficiency of vitamin B_6

Deficiency of vitamin B_6 due to inadequate intake from the diet is rare, although alcoholics are at a higher risk due to low intake and impaired metabolism of the vitamin. Deprivation of vitamin B_6 leads to metabolic abnormalities resulting from insufficient production of PLP. The deficiency manifests clinically as dermatologic and neurologic changes. Humans show symptoms of weakness, irritability, sleeplessness, peripheral neuropathy, cheilosis (lips become dry and chaffed), glossitis (tongue becomes red and shiny), stomatitis (angles at the corners of the mouth become ulcerated). Advanced symptoms include growth failure, impaired motor function, and convulsions. Immune function is also impaired in vitamin B_6 deficiency.

Due to the widespread distribution of vitamin B_6 in foods, cases of deficiency are rare. However, deficiency may be precipitated by certain medications. One example is a drug called Isonicotinic Acid Hydrazide (INH) which is widely used in the treatment of tuberculosis. INH acts as an antagonist to vitamin B_6 and patients who have been treated with INH often develop deficiency symptoms.

Pregnant women and women using oral contraceptive pills also have increased requirements of this vitamin, and they are at higher risk of deficiency.

Vitamin B_6 deficiency has also been observed in infants who have been fed synthetic milk or food lacking in vitamin B_6. The infants showed nervous irritability and convulsive seizures. The convulsions respond dramatically to supplements of vitamin B_6.

Vitamin B_6 toxicity

Acute toxicity of vitamin B_6 is rare. However, when it is taken in pharmacologic doses, as in therapy for premenstrual syndrome, toxic effects can be produced. Toxicity symptoms include depression, fatigue, irritability, headaches and lack of muscle coordination, nerve damage causing numbness and muscle weakness leading to inability to walk. Megadoses of vitamins should be used with caution. Because of interrelationships in metabolism of various nutrients, mega dose of a vitamin can induce deficiency of other vitamins.

Pantothenic Acid

Pantothenic acid is a water-soluble B-complex vitamin. It was isolated in 1938 by Dr. R J Williams. However, its role as a coenzyme was elucidated in 1946. Pantothenic acid is widely distributed in foods and in body tissues. In fact, it derives its name from the Greek word *panthos* meaning 'everywhere'.

Most foods contain pantothenic acid in its coenzyme form, which is digested in the intestine to release the free vitamin. The latter is absorbed from the small intestine and transported to various body tissues in the free form. Within the tissues, pantothenic acid is converted to the coenzyme form. It is widely distributed in most body tissues, particularly the liver, kidney, brain, heart, adrenals and testes.

Pantothenic acid is highly soluble in water. There is little loss of the vitamin in ordinary cooking procedures except in acidic and alkaline solutions. There is no known toxicity of the vitamin nor a natural deficiency state.

Functions of pantothenic acid

Pantothenic acid acts as a component of coenzymes that are involved in more than 100 different metabolic reactions that sustain life. Pantothenic acid functions in the body as a component of Coenzyme A (CoA) and Acyl Carrier Protein (ACP). In these forms, pantothenic acid is essential for the metabolism of fatty acids, amino acids, and carbohydrates. It catalyses important metabolic reactions that generate energy from food (fat, carbohydrates and proteins).

Both CoA and ACP function in our body as carriers of acyl group. CoA functions in reactions that accept or remove the acetyl group ($-CH_3CO$). Some of the important reactions in which CoA is involved are explained here.

- In the formation of acetylcholine, a substance in the transmission of nerve impulses
- In important catabolic reactions such as oxidation of glucose and fatty acids that generate energy
- In the synthesis of cholesterol and other sterols in the body
- In the synthesis of porphyrin, a component of haemoglobin
- Both CoA and ACP are required for the synthesis of fatty acids in the body

Daily allowances of pantothenic acid

Since pantothenic acid is widespread in foods and its deficiency is unknown, a quantitative requirement for pantothenic acid has not been established. ICMR has not established a level of RDA for our Indian population. The Food and Nutrition Board in the United States too has not established its RDA but they have suggested a level of Adequate Intake (AI) of pantothenic acid for different age groups. Their recommendations have been given in table 13.

Table 13
Recommended intake of pantothenic acid (mg/day)

Group	Age	Males	Females
Infants	0-6 months	1.7	1.7
Infants	7-12 months	1.8	1.8
Children	1-3 years	2	2
Children	4-8 years	3	3
Children	9-13 years	4	4
Adolescents	14-18 years	5	5
Adults	-	5	5
Pregnant women	-	-	6
Lactating women	-	-	7

Rich sources of pantothenic acid

Pantothenic acid is present in both plant and animal foods. Rich sources include liver, kidney, yeast, egg yolk and broccoli. Among the more commonly consumed foods chicken, fish, milk, curd, legumes, mushrooms and sweet potatoes are good sources. Whole grain cereals are also good sources of pantothenic acid. However, most of it is located in the outer layers of the grain and about half the vitamin is lost during milling.

Pantothenic acid content of Indian foods has not been extensively studied. Wheat and jowar contain about 1-1.5mg/100g, and milk contains about 0.4mg/100g. Ordinary Indian diets provide about 5-10mg, which is usually adequate since deficiency is rare. Pantothenic acid content of selected foods in western diets is given in table 14.

Table 14
Pantothenic acid content in certain food items

Foodstuff	Pantothenic acid (mg)
Bread, whole wheat, 1 slice	0.18
Soyabean flour, ½ cup	1.00
Wheat germ, ¼ cup	0.39
Broccoli, raw, ½ cup	0.24
Corn, yellow, boiled, ½ cup	0.72
Potato, baked, 1 medium	1.12
Sweet potato, boiled, ½ cup	0.87
Tomato, boiled, ½ cup	0.35
Apricot, 3 medium	0.25
Banana, 1 medium	0.30
Orange juice, 1 cup	0.47
Papaya, 1 medium	0.66

Foodstuff	Pantothenic acid (mg)
Pomegranate, 1 medium	0.92
Beef, liver, 3.5 ounce	5.92
Chicken, 3.5 ounce	0.97
Egg, 1 large	0.86
Egg yolk, 1	0.75
Peanut, roasted, 1 ounce	0.39
Almond, 1 ounce	0.13
Cashew nut, 1 ounce	0.34
Lentil, boiled, ½ cup	0.63
Milk, skimmed, 1 cup	0.81
Milk, whole, 1 cup	0.76
Cheddar cheese, 1 ounce	0.12
Curd, 1 cup	0.88

Deficiency of pantothenic acid

Naturally occurring pantothenic acid deficiency in humans is rare. However when deficient diets were fed to volunteers along with an antagonist the following symptoms were observed – loss of appetite, indigestion, abdominal pain, headache, fatigue, mental depression, sleeplessness, numbness and tingling of hands and feet.

Biotin

Biotin is a water-soluble vitamin, generally classified as a B-complex vitamin. Biotin was first isolated in 1936 and synthesised in 1943. Dr. Helen Parsons observed symptoms such as eczema and hair loss in rats being fed a diet including raw egg white. The symptoms were cured by adding egg yolk to the diet of the affected animals. The corrective factor was isolated and termed 'biotin'.

The substance in raw egg white was identified to be a biotin antagonist, which prevented its absorption. The substance was called avidin and it could be easily destroyed by heat.

Biotin is required by all organisms but can only be synthesised by bacteria, yeast, molds, algae and some plants. The bacteria in our intestinal tract also synthesise biotin, which can be absorbed in parts from the intestinal tract. Biotin is stored in minute amounts in the metabolically active tissues such as the kidney, liver, brain and adrenal. There are no known toxic effects from biotin.

A relatively simple compound, soluble in water, biotin is stable to heat, light and acids, but somewhat sensitive to alkalis and oxidising agents. In tissues and in foods, it is usually combined with protein.

Functions of biotin

Biotin plays an important role in metabolism as a coenzyme that carries carbon dioxide. This role is critical in the energy cycle in carboxylation and decarboxylation reactions. It participates in carbon dioxide fixation reactions that transfer carbon dioxide from one compound to another. In the energy cycle, biotin fixes carbon dioxide on to a 3-carbon compound to form a 4-carbon compound, which keeps the energy cycle going. It is required in the energy cycle and is thus essential for the production of energy from glucose. Carboxylation reactions involving biotin are also a part of the following metabolic pathways:

- Synthesis of fatty acids
- Breakdown of fats and amino acids to form glucose
- Metabolism of amino acids and cholesterol
- Synthesis of some components of DNA and RNA

Biotin is thus essential for the metabolism of carbohydrates, fats and proteins, as well as nucleic acids such as DNA and RNA.

Daily allowances of biotin

Since the amount of biotin needed for metabolism is minute, its requirement has not been established in specific terms. Indian data on biotin requirements, contents in foodstuffs, and intestinal synthesis of biotin is limited and deficiency of biotin is rare. Hence, ICMR has not established RDA for biotin for Indian population.

The Food and Nutrition Board in the United States also felt that the available data was insufficient to calculate an RDA for biotin, so they set an Adequate Intake (AI) level for biotin for different age groups. Their recommendations have been given in table 15.

Table 15
Recommended intake of biotin (mg/day)

Group	Age	Males	Females
Infants	0-6 months	5	5
Infants	7-12 months	6	6
Children	1-3 years	8	8
Children	4-8 years	12	12
Children	9-13 years	20	20
Adolescents	14-18 years	25	25
Adults	-	30	30
Pregnant women	-	-	30
Lactating women	-	-	35

Rich sources of biotin

Biotin is widely distributed in foods but few foods have high concentrations. Milk, liver, egg yolk, legumes, nuts and a few vegetables are the most important sources of biotin in human diets. The bioavailability of biotin varies considerably among different foods. This is because biotin is bound to protein to form complexes in different foods. The availability of biotin from these complexes depends upon the digestibility of that complex.

The availability of biotin from raw egg presents a typical case of protein-biotin complexes, which led to its discovery. Egg white contains a protein called avidin (antivitamin). Avidin binds biotin to form a complex, which is resistant to digestion. Biotin from raw egg is thus not available to the body. Cooking denatures avidin and inactivates its biotin-binding capacity. Biotin from cooked eggs is easily absorbed from the intestine.

The bacteria present in the large intestine of human beings are capable of synthesising biotin, which can be assimilated by the body from the large intestine. The bioavailability of this biotin is variable but usually is considered sufficient because biotin is rare.

Indian data on biotin content of foodstuffs is limited. Biotin content of selected foods in western diets is listed in table 16.

Table 16
Biotin content in certain food items

Foodstuff	Biotin (mg/100g)
Wheat germ	22-38
Wheat bran	22.4-25.5
Oatmeal, rolled oats	15.3-24.6
Milk, whole	1.6-2.4
Milk, human	18-22
Egg, cooked	20-25
Egg yolk, raw	515-58
Chicken, liver	170-210
Beef, liver	96
Poultry	10-11.3
Fish and shellfish	3-24
Vegetable	0.2-4.1
Fruit	0.2-2
Almond, raw	18
Peanut, roasted	34
Chocolate	32

Deficiency of biotin

Since biotin is widespread in foods — it is also available from intestinal synthesis, and the requirement is minute — natural biotin deficiency is rare. However, biotin deficiency can be induced by feeding large quantities of raw egg white which contains avidin, a protein that binds biotin and prevents its absorption in the body. Cooking the egg white inactivates avidin. Therefore, consumption of cooked egg has no effect on biotin absorption in the body. Symptoms of deficiency include loss of appetite, nausea, hair loss, and scaly red rash around the eyes, nose, mouth and genital area. Neurological symptoms include depression, lethargy, hallucination and numbness and tingling sensation in the hands and feet.

Folic Acid

Folic acid, also known as folacin or folate is a water-soluble B-complex vitamin. It was described by several researchers during the 1930s and 1940s as a factor required by some animals. Folic acid was named in 1941 by Mitchell; its name is derived from the Latin word for leaf, *'folium'* due to its widespread prevalence in green leafy vegetables and its acidic nature.

The chemical name of folic acid is pteryolglutamic acid. It is composed of three acids – Pteroic Acid, Para-aminobenzoic Acid (PABA) and Glutamic Acid. About 25% of the folacin in foods is in the free form and is readily absorbed. The rest is conjugated with additional glutamic acid groups. This needs to be digested before absorption. The bioavailability of folates from diet is only about 50%.

Folacin is stored principally in the liver. The coenzyme form of folic acid is Tetrahydrofolic Acid (THF). Vitamin C prevents the oxidation of this active form of folic acid, which functions as a coenzyme in several reactions.

Folic acid is sparingly soluble in water and stable in alkalis. It is easily oxidised in acidic medium and is sensitive to light. No adverse effects of high oral doses of folate have been reported.

Functions of folic acid

Folates function as coenzymes that link up with and transfer single-carbon units in a variety of metabolic reactions involving nucleic acids and amino acids. A number of key compounds are formed as a result of this transfer. One of these is THF. Together with vitamin B_{12}, THF is essential for the synthesis of nitrogen-containing compounds, purines and pyrimidines, which are the building blocks of DNA and RNA. DNA and RNA are the information molecules of our body, which carry all the genetic information. Another important function of folic acid is in the synthesis of haeme, the iron-containing part of haemoglobin. Folic acid is thus necessary for the synthesis and maturation of Red Blood Cells (RBCs). Because of its role in DNA synthesis and RBC formation, folate requirements increase during periods of accelerated growth such as pregnancy, lactation and adolescence.

Folate enzymes are also required for the synthesis of several important amino acids. It is required for the synthesis of amino acid serine and for the conversion of homocysteine to amino acid methionine. Folate deficiency can result in decreased synthesis of methionine and increased levels of homocysteine. The latter is a risk factor for heart disease.

Because folacin is required for protein synthesis, folacin inhibitors have been successfully used in the chemotherapy of various types of cancer.

In many of its functions, folic acid is associated with vitamin B_{12}. Vitamin B_{12} also makes available the active form of the folate coenzymes to participate in purine and pyrimidine synthesis and other functions.

Daily allowances of folic acid

The bioavailability of folate is only about 50% from an average diet. This is because part of the folic acid is in conjugated form. Some losses also occur during cooking. The ICMR has established the RDA for folic acid for Indian population keeping in mind the bioavailability of folic acid from diets.

Requirements of folic acid increase considerably during growth periods such as pregnancy, lactation and adolescence. The folic acid requirements for different age groups, activity level, sex, and physiological groups, as per the recommendations of ICMR are given in table 17.

Table 17
Recommended intake of folic acid (mg/day)

Group	Age	Males	Females
Infants	0-12 months	25	25
Children	1-3 years	30	30
Children	4-6 years	40	40
Children	7-9 years	60	60
Children	10-12 years	70	70
Adolescents	13-15 years	100	100
Adolescents	16-18 years	100	100
Adults	-	100	100
Pregnant women	-	-	400
Lactating women	-	-	150

Rich sources of folic acid

Folates occur in a variety of foods of both plant and animal origins in both free and conjugated form. The free form can be readily absorbed. However, the conjugated form first needs to be released before absorption and its availability to meet the body needs is unknown.

Folates are especially abundant in green leafy vegetables and legumes. The vitamin's name suggests the word *foliage*, and indeed, green leafy vegetables (especially spinach and broccoli) are outstanding sources. Liver, kidney, yeast and mushrooms too are excellent sources. Lean beef, egg, whole-grain cereals, potatoes and dried beans are also good sources. However, most root vegetables, milk and milk products, light green vegetables and meats are relatively low in folic acid.

Heat and oxidation during cooking can destroy as much as half of the folate in foods. The bioavailability of folates in foods depends upon a number of factors such as form of the vitamin (free/conjugate) and nutritional status of the person (deficiency of iron and vitamin C can impair utilisation of folic acid). The bioavailability of folic acid supplement is 100% if the stomach is empty.

The folic acid content (both free and total) of commonly consumed foods is given in Appendix II.

Deficiency of folic acid

Folate deficiency impairs cell division and protein synthesis, both of which are critical to growing tissues. The deficiency is most apparent in cells with rapid multiplication, such as RBCs, WBCs and epithelial cells of the stomach and intestine. In folate deficiency, the replacement of red blood cells and gastrointestinal tract cells falter. Two of the first symptoms of folate deficiency are anaemia and gastrointestinal tract deterioration.

Anaemia due to folate deficiency is called megaloblastic anaemia. It is characterised by large, immature blood cells. With the absence of folate,

DNA synthesis slows down and the cells lose their ability to divide. As a result, the immature blood cells are enlarged and oval-shaped. They cannot carry oxygen to the tissues or travel through the capillaries as efficiently as normal RBCs. This results in symptoms such as fatigue, weakness, and shortness of breath.

The deterioration of the gastrointestinal tract due to folate deficiency results in a vicious cycle because the deteriorated gastrointestinal tract is unable to absorb any nutrients.

Folate deficiency can occur in a number of situations. For example, low dietary intake and diminished absorption, as in alcoholism, can result in a decreased supply of folate. Folate deficiency can develop from inadequate intake in infants fed on goat's milk, which is very low in folate. Folate requirements increase considerably during pregnancy. A deficiency of folic acid during the early weeks of pregnancy may result in various central nervous system disorders called neural tube defects and even death.

Folate deficiency can also develop deficiency of another nutrient. As mentioned earlier, the metabolism of folic acid and vitamin B_{12} are linked. The folate coenzyme is attached to a methyl group (CH_3) while it is being transported in the body. To function as a coenzyme, the methyl group must be removed. The enzyme that removes the methyl group requires the help of vitamin B_{12}. Without vitamin B_{12}, folate becomes trapped and unable to perform its functions resulting in a functional deficiency. Heavy use of drugs such as aspirins and antacids, oral contraceptive pills and smoking also interferes with the body's handling of folate.

Vitamin B_{12}

Vitamin B_{12} is the largest and most complex of all the vitamins. It is unique among vitamins in that it contains a metal ion, cobalt. For this reason, compounds with vitamin B_{12} activity are referred to as 'cobalamins'. Vitamin B_{12}, isolated in 1948 from liver extract, was the last vitamin to be identified. The structure of this complex vitamin was elucidated in 1955.

Vitamin B_{12} occurs in several forms. Cyanocobalamin, the form available commercially, is the most stable form. Forms found in body tissues include methylcobalamin, hydroxycobalamin and adenosylcobalamin.

Vitamin B_{12} is different from most other vitamins in that its only source in nature is microbial synthesis. It is not found in any plant foods, but it is widely distributed in animal tissues.

Absorption of vitamin B_{12} is unique among vitamins in that it requires an 'intrinsic factor' for absorption. This factor is necessary to carry the vitamin across the walls of the intestine and into the blood stream. In adequately nourished individuals, vitamin B_{12} is stored in appreciable amounts (approximately 2000mg), mainly in the liver, which typically accumulates a substantial store, some 5 to 7 years worth. There are no known toxic effects from daily oral doses of up to 100mg (100 times the RDA).

Vitamin B_{12} is slightly soluble in water, stable to heat, but inactivated by light and by strong acids and alkalis. Excessive amounts of vitamin C present in a meal may lead to destruction of vitamin B_{12}. There is little loss of vitamin B_{12} in food during ordinary cooking procedures.

Functions of vitamin B_{12}

Vitamin B_{12} acts as a coenzyme in methylation reactions. Methylation reactions involve the transfer of methyl groups (CH_3) from one compound to another. Although vitamin B_{12} performs its methylation task in only two reactions, these reactions are critical in metabolism.

In the first reaction, methylcobalamin acts as a coenzyme in the conversion of homocysteine to methionine. This reaction is accompanied by the conversion of methyl-tetrahydrofolate to tetrahydrofolate. Methionine is an essential amino acid, which participates in the synthesis of DNA and RNA. This reaction also regenerates the active forms of the folate and vitamin B_{12} coenzymes.

Adenosylcobalamin acts as a coenzyme in the conversion of methylmalonyl-CoA to succinyl-CoA. This biochemical reaction plays an important role in the production of energy from fats and proteins.

Vitamin B_{12} is also critical to the central nervous system. It maintains the sheath that surrounds and protects nerve fibres and promotes their normal growth.

Since vitamin B_{12} shares a close metabolic interrelationship with folic acid, it is indirectly involved in the formation of RBCs.

Daily allowances of vitamin B_{12}

The amount of dietary vitamin B_{12} that is required for normal human metabolism appears to be small. The micro-organisms present in our large intestine are capable of synthesising vitamin B_{12} but whether this vitamin is available for absorption is not known for sure. The ICMR has established the RDA for vitamin B_{12} for Indian population. The requirements vary depending upon age and physiological conditions. The RDA for vitamin B_{12} are given in table 18.

Table 18
Recommended intake of vitamin B_{12} (mg/day)

Group	Age	Males	Females
Infants	0-12 months	0.2	0.2
Children	1-3 years	0.2-1.0	0.2-1.0
Children	4-6 years	0.2-1.0	0.2-1.0
Children	7-9 years	0.2-1.0	0.2-1.0
Children	10-12 years	0.2-1.0	0.2-1.0
Adolescents	13-15 years	0.2-1.0	0.2-1.0
Adolescents	16-18 years	0.2-1.0	0.2-1.0
Adults	-	1	1
Pregnant women	-	-	1
Lactating women	-	-	1.5

Rich sources of vitamin B_{12}

Vitamin B_{12} is unique among the vitamins in being found almost exclusively in foods derived from animals. This reason is that vitamin B_{12} can be synthesised only by some microorganisms including bacteria. The bacteria in the large intestine of human beings are also capable of synthesising vitamin B_{12}, although we cannot utilise the vitamin from this source.

The richest sources of vitamin B_{12} are liver, kidney, milk, eggs, fish, cheese, meats and poultry. Foods of plant origin may also contain vitamin B_{12} from bacterial contamination. Natural dietary deficiency is rare, and is observed only in strict vegetarians who do not consume any animal products, including milk. People not taking food containing B_{12} may take up to 20 years to develop deficiency because the body recycles much of its vitamin B_{12} and reuses it over and over again.

Approximately 70% of the vitamin activity is retained during cooking of most foods. However, vitamin B_{12} can be lost during pasteurisation of milk and during microwave cooking.

Indian data on vitamin B_{12} content of foods is unavailable. Vitamin B_{12} content of selected foods in western diets is given in table 19.

Table 19
Vitamin B12 content in certain food items

Foodstuff	Vitamin B_{12} (mg)
Beef, liver, fried, 3.5 ounce	111.80
Chicken, liver, 3.5 ounce	19.39
Chicken, roasted, 3.5 ounce	0.34
Egg, fresh, 1 large	0.77
Ham, regular, 3.5 ounce	0.80
Salmon, baked, 3 ounce	4.93
Milk, skimmed, 1 cup	0.93
Milk, whole, 1 cup	0.87
Full cream milk curd, 1 cup	0.84
Cheddar cheese, 3.5 ounce	0.83

Deficiency of vitamin B_{12}

Vitamin B_{12} deficiency is clinically known as pernicious anaemia. Vitamin B_{12} deficiency results in the impairment of the activity of the enzymes requiring vitamin B_{12}. There is an elevation in the levels of the metabolites, homocysteine and methylmalonyl-CoA. Elevated blood levels of homocysteine are an independent risk factor for heart disease.

The reaction involving homocysteine also results in the regeneration of the active form of the folate coenzyme. As a result of vitamin B_{12} deficiency, folate gets trapped in the inactive form, creating a functional folate deficiency. Thus, in both folate and vitamin B_{12} deficiency, folate is unavailable to participate in DNA synthesis. This impairment of DNA synthesis affects the rapidly dividing cells of the bone marrow (where RBCs are produced). The result is the production of large, immature RBCs, which are not capable of carrying oxygen.

Deficiency of vitamin B_{12} also results in neurological symptoms such as numbness and tingling of the arms and legs, difficulty in walking, amnesia, depression, disorientation and dementia, with or without mood swings. The progression of the neurological complications is gradual. Vitamin B_{12} deficiency is known to damage the myelin sheath covering the nerves in the brain and spinal cord.

The megaloblastic anaemia of folate deficiency is similar to that of vitamin B_{12} deficiency. However, if the anaemia resulting from folate deficiency, is cured with folate, the anaemia would be cured, but the neurological symptoms would persist. Megaloblastic anaemia should not be treated with folate unless the underlying cause of deficiency is known.

Vitamin B_{12} deficiency due to inadequate diet intake is rare because the requirement is minute, and even most pure vegetarians manage to obtain sufficient amounts due to bacterial contamination of plant foods. Vitamin B_{12} deficiency usually occurs due to a defect in absorption. It requires an intrinsic factor for absorption; any condition resulting in defective intrinsic factor production can result in vitamin B_{12} deficiency. A patient suffering from defective vitamin B_{12} absorption needs to be given injections of the vitamin to bypass the intestinal absorption route.

Vitamin C

Vitamin C, also known as ascorbic acid, is the antiscorbutic factor. It is a water-soluble vitamin, which is essential for the normal functioning of the body. Unlike most mammals, human beings do not have the ability to make their own vitamin C. We must therefore, obtain it from the diet.

Scurvy had been known as a dreaded disease since ancient times. In 1747, Dr. James Lind, a British physician, found that oranges and lemons could cure scurvy. During the same period, Captain Cook was able to reduce the incidence of scurvy on his ongoing voyages by stocking up fresh fruits and vegetables. The antiscorbutic factor was isolated in 1928 by Dr. Szent-Gyorgyi and its chemical structure was elucidated by him and Dr. C G King in 1932.

Of all the water-soluble vitamins, vitamin C is the most unstable and easily destroyed vitamin. It is highly soluble in water and gets easily destroyed by oxygen, alkalis and high temperature. Vitamin C is easily oxidised to dehydroascorbic acid, which is also active. The oxidation is accelerated by heat, light, alkalis, oxidative enzymes and traces of metals such as copper and iron. Oxidation is inhibited to a marked degree in an acid reaction and when the temperature is reduced. Vitamin C is easily destroyed during cooking.

On an average, about 50% of the vitamin C in foods is lost during different cooking procedures, although these could be higher than the quoted figure. On the contrary, fermentation and germination result in significant increase in the vitamin C content of foodstuffs.

Functions of vitamin C

Vitamin C serves several metabolic functions – as an enzyme cofactor, an antioxidant, a protective agent, and as a reactant with transition metal ions. Each of these functions involves the oxidation/reduction properties of the vitamin. Vitamin C is easily oxidised and this forms the basis of most of its functions in the body.

The first step in the formation of bone is a fibrous network, which consists largely of a protein called collagen. More generally speaking, collagen is found in the 'connective tissue' or the tissue, which holds together different tissues or organs, including the walls of the blood vessels. One of the principal functions of vitamin C is in the formation of collagen. In the synthesis of collagen, vitamin C is essential for the hydroxylation (addition of -OH groups) of amino acids – proline and lysine. The hydroxyamino acids – hydroxyproline and hydroxylysine – are essential constituents of collagen. Thus, vitamin C is important in the healing of wounds and fractures, and in maintaining the integrity of blood capillaries.

Vitamin C also plays an important role in other hydroxylation reactions. These involve the conversion of amino acid tryptophan to serotonin, an important neurotransmitter, and the conversion of amino acid tyrosine to norepinephrine. Vitamin C is also required for the breakdown of cholesterol to bile acids.

Vitamin C is required for the conversion of folacin to tetrahydrofolic acid, the active form of the vitamin. Vitamin C also enhances the absorption of iron by reducing the ferric ion to ferrous. It also promotes resistance to infections through the immunologic activity of leukocytes (white blood cells).

Vitamin C is an important antioxidant and thus has a role in the protection of vitamins A and E and polyunsaturated fatty acids from excessive oxidation. By virtue of its antioxidant property, vitamin C can quench potentially toxic reactive species (free radicals) from causing oxidative damage to body tissues.

Daily allowances of vitamin C

The minimum amount of vitamin C required to prevent scurvy is only 10mg per day. However, at this level of intake, the body tissues are not saturated with vitamin C. At an intake of 20mg per day, the level of vitamin C in body tissues becomes satisfactory. Since vitamin C is extremely heat-labile, cooking losses of vitamin C have to be considered in determining the RDA. On an average, 50% of the vitamin content of raw foods is lost during cooking and storage. Hence, ICMR has recommended a daily allowance of 40mg per day for adults. The recommendations of ICMR for different age groups are given in table 20.

Table 20
Recommended intake of vitamin C (mg/day)

Group	Age	Males	Females
Infants	0-12 months	25	25
Children	1-3 years	40	40
Children	4-6 years	40	40
Children	7-9 years	40	40
Children	10-12 years	40	40
Adolescents	13-15 years	40	40
Adolescents	16-18 years	40	40
Adults	-	40	40
Pregnant women	-	-	40
Lactating women	-	-	80

Certain stress conditions such as infections, burns, extremes of temperatures, intake of toxic metals, chronic use of medications such as aspirin, and oral contraceptives, and cigarette smoking are known to increase vitamin C requirements. Cigarette smoke contains oxidants, which deplete vitamin C from the body. The Food and Nutrition Board in the United States has recommended an intake of at least 100mg of vitamin C per day for cigarette smokers.

Rich sources of vitamin C

Almost all the daily intake of vitamin C is obtained from fruits and vegetables. Vitamin C is often called the 'fresh-food vitamin', since it is found in highest concentrations when the food is fresh from the plant.

Citrus fruits such as oranges, lemon, mausambi and grapefruit are excellent sources of vitamin C. Orange sections, including the thin white peel, contain more vitamin C than an equal weight of strained juices. Amla (the Indian gooseberry) and guava are among the cheapest and best sources of vitamin C. Fresh strawberries, papaya and pineapple are also good sources of vitamin C. Other non-acid fruits such as peaches, pears, bananas and sapota (*chikoo*) are also fair sources and can make an important contribution to the diet.

Broccoli, spinach, cabbage, turnips and brussels sprouts are excellent-to-good sources even when cooked. Potato can also be an important source of vitamin C if it is used as a staple food.

Milk (except breast milk), eggs, meat, fish and chicken are practically devoid of vitamin C. If the mother's diet is adequate, human milk contains 4 to 6 times as much vitamin C as in cow's milk and is able to protect infants from scurvy. Liver contains a small amount of vitamin C, most of which is lost during cooking. The vitamin C content of commonly consumed foods is given in Appendix II.

Dry cereals and legumes contain small amounts (1-8mg/100g) of vitamin C which increase enormously during germination. Sprouted cereals contain 5-10mg whereas sprouted pulses contain 50-75mg vitamin C per 100g. Fermentation also results in significant increase in vitamin C content of foodstuffs. Some foods such as amla, mango and chillies retain their vitamin C activity even in the dry form.

Retention of vitamin C during cooking

The loss of vitamin C during cooking depends on the method employed. The loss can be minimised by using the right cooking techniques. Vegetables should be cooked rapidly under cover to minimise the time and degree of exposure to air. The losses are less when they are cut into larger pieces than when they are finely chopped. Cooking along with pulses, addition of tamarind juice, lemon juice, or sour buttermilk during cooking or even towards the end of cooking, reduces losses as an acid medium prevents oxidation. Root vegetables and tubers such as potatoes should be boiled along with their skin to reduce losses. The vegetables should be washed well before peeling or cutting and they should be cut right before cooking to avoid exposure to air. The surplus water used in cooking should be used in soups or gravy.

Deficiency of vitamin C

A deficiency of vitamin C impairs collagen formation and retards healing of bone fractures. Two of the most notable signs of vitamin C deficiency reflect its role in maintaining the integrity of blood vessels. The gums bleed easily around the teeth and capillaries under the skin break spontaneously, producing pinpoint haemorrhages.

The first symptoms of scurvy include weakness, fatigue, loss of appetite, depression, and swollen gums, which bleed profusely on touching. Muscles, including the heart muscle, begin to degenerate. The skin becomes rough, brown, scaly and dry. Wounds fail to heal as scar tissue does not form. Bone rebuilding falters; the ends of long bones become softened, malformed, painful and prone to fractures. The joints become swollen and painful. Since vitamin C is involved in iron metabolism, anaemia is often associated with scurvy.

Vitamin C toxicity

The easy availability of vitamin C supplements and publication of materials claiming that vitamin C is a cure for colds and cancers have led thousands of people to take large doses of vitamin C. The main adverse effects produced due to excessive vitamin C intake include nausea, abdominal cramps, and diarrhoea. Another toxic effect could be the formation of oxalate stones in kidney because the breakdown of vitamin C yields oxalates. Vitamin C supplements are toxic for people with iron overload because it promotes iron absorption. An upper intake level of 2g vitamin C per day has been suggested to prevent gastrointestinal disturbances from excessive intakes.

Myths and Facts

Myth
Vitamin pills containing 10 times the RDA are a better buy.

Fact
Only the recommended allowances of various nutrients should be consumed unless special conditions such as a deficiency or disease exists.

Myth
Everyone should take vitamin pills.

Fact
Healthy individuals do not need vitamin supplements if they eat a well-balanced diet from the basic food groups.

Myth
Expensive vitamins provide superior nutrients resulting in better health.

Fact

Higher prices of vitamin pills are related to sales promotion and advertising. The cost of the chemicals in the pill is usually very small. A wise customer should buy the amount and type of pill desired, which can be established by reading the label and composition.

Myth

Only natural vitamins should be taken.

Fact

Vitamins are chemical substances occurring naturally in foods, but the same chemical compound synthesised in a laboratory performs in exactly the same way as the natural food source vitamin. The chemical structures of all vitamins have been identified and the synthetic vitamins are identical in structure and function to the natural vitamins. One advantage of a synthetic vitamin is that it is usually more compact and smaller in size. In some cases, the natural form of a vitamin is less potent (folic acid) or more susceptible to degradation (vitamin E). The forms of niacin and vitamin B_6 in supplements and additives are more efficiently utilised than the forms found in whole grain cereals.

Myth
A tired feeling without as much energy as desired, implies the need for vitamin supplementation.

Fact
There are many nutrients that produce energy. In fact, almost all the known nutrients have at least an indirect effect on how energetic a person is. Even those that are identified as directly involved in energy production, such as carbohydrates, iron, and B vitamins, cannot be used by the body without many other nutrients. A strange phenomenon can occur with megadoses of many nutrients. As has been mentioned in various sections of the book, excessive intake of vitamins can produce toxicity symptoms, some of which are similar to deficiency symptoms. For example fatigue, which is a symptom of many deficiency diseases, can also be caused by a self-medicated overdose. The wisest advise for fatigue is to ensure a well-balanced diet under leisurely conditions, regular outdoor activity, and adequate rest. If fatigue continues, laboratory assessment should be ordered.

Appendix I
Recommended Dietary Allowances

Group	Age	Body wt. kg	Net energy Cal/d	Protein g/d	Fat g/d	Calcium mg/d	Iron mg/d	Vitamin A µg/d Retinol	Vitamin A µg/d B carotene	Thiamin Carotene	Riboflavin mg/d	Niacin oxine mg/d	Yrid mg/d	Vit. C mg/d	Folic acid µg/d	Vit. B₁₂ µg/d
Men	Sedentary	60	2425	-	-	-	-	-	-	1.2	1.4	16	-	-	-	-
	Moderate	60	2875	60	20	400	28	600	2400	1.4	1.6	18	2.0	40	100	1
	Heavy	60	3800	-	-	-	-	-	-	1.6	1.9	21	-	-	-	-
Women	Sedentary	50	1875	-	-	-	-	-	-	0.9	1.1	12	-	-	-	-
	Moderate	50	2225	50	20	400	30	600	2400	1.1	1.3	14	2.0	40	100	1
	Heavy	50	2925	-	-	-	-	-	-	1.2	1.5	16	-	-	-	1
	Pregnant	-	+300	+15	30	1000	38	600	2400	+0.2	+0.2	+2	2.5	40	400	1
	Lactating 0-6 mths.	-	+550	+25	45	1000	30	950	3800	+0.3	+0.3	+4	2.5	80	150	1.5
	6-12 mths.	-	+400	+18	45	1000	30	950	3800	+0.2	+0.2	+3	2.5	80	150	1.5
Infants	0-6 mths.	5.4	108 /kg	2.05 /kg	-	500	-	350	1400	55 µg/kg	65 µg/kg	710 µg/kg	0.1	25	25	0.2
	6-12 mths.	8.6	98 /kg	1.65 /kg	-	500	-	350	1400	50 µg/kg	60 µg/kg	650 µg/kg	0.4	25	25	0.2
Children	1-3	12.2	1240	22	-	-	12	400	1600	0.6	0.7	8	0.9	-	30	-
	4-6	19.0	1690	30	25	400	18	400	1600	0.9	1.0	11	0.9	40	40	0.2-
	7-9	26.9	1950	41	-	-	26	600	2400	1.0	1.2	13	1.6	-	60	1.0
Boys	10-12	35.4	2190	54	25	600	34	600	2400	1.1	1.3	15	1.6	40	70	0.2-
Girls	10-12	31.5	1970	57	25	600	19	600	2400	1.0	1.2	13	1.6	40	70	1.0
Boys	13-15	47.8	2450	70	25	600	41	600	2400	1.2	1.5	16	2.0	40	100	0.2-
Girls	13-15	46.7	2060	65	25	600	28	600	2400	1.0	1.2	14	2.0	40	100	1.0
Boys	16-18	57.1	2640	78	25	500	50	600	2400	1.3	1.6	17	2.0	40	100	0.2-
Girls	16-18	49.9	2060	63	25	500	30	600	2400	1.0	1.2	14	2.0	40	100	1.0

Source: Indian Council of Medical Research, 1996 (reprint)

Appendix II
Vitamin Content of Common Foods
(All the values are per 100g of edible portion)

Foodstuff	Carotene (µg)	Thiamin (mg)	Riboflavin (mg)	Niacin (mg)	Vitamin B_6 (mg)	Folic acid(µg) Free	Folic acid(µg) Total	Vitamin C (mg)
Cereal, grains and products								
Bajra	132	0.33	0.25	2.3	-	14.7	45.5	0
Barley	10	0.47	0.20	5.4	-	-	-	0
Jowar	47	0.37	0.13	3.1	0.21	14.0	20.0	0
Maize, dry	90	0.42	0.10	1.8	-	14.0	20.0	0
Rice, milled, parboiled	-	0.21	0.05	3.8	0.24	8.9	11.0	0
Rice, milled, raw	0	0.06	0.06	1.9	-	4.1	8.0	0
Rice, flaked	0	0.21	0.05	4.0	-	-	-	0
Rice, puffed	0	0.21	0.01	4.1	-	-	-	0
Wheat, flour (whole)	29	0.49	0.17	4.3	-	12.1	35.8	0
Wheat, flour (refined)	25	0.12	0.07	2.4	-	-	-	0
Wheat, semolina	-	0.12	0.03	1.6	-	-	-	0
Wheat, vermicelli	0	0.19	0.05	1.8	-	-	-	0
Wheat, bread (brown)	-	0.21	-	2.5	-	-	-	-
Wheat, bread (white)	-	0.07	-	0.7	-	-	-	-
Pulses and legumes								
Bengal gram, whole	189	0.30	0.15	2.9	-	34.0	186.0	3
Bengal gram, dal	129	0.48	0.18	2.4	-	32.0	147.5	1
Bengal gram, roasted	113	0.20	-	1.3	-	22.0	139.0	0
Black gram, dal	38	0.42	0.20	2.0	-	24.0	132.0	0
Cow pea	12	0.51	0.20	1.3	-	69.0	133.0	0
Green gram, whole	94	0.47	0.27	2.1	-	-	-	0
Green gram, dal	49	0.47	0.21	2.4	-	24.5	140.0	0
Lentil	270	0.45	0.20	2.6	-	14.5	36.0	0
Pea, green	83	0.25	0.01	0.8	-	-	-	9
Pea, dry	39	0.47	0.19	3.4	-	4.6	7.5	0
Red gram, dal	132	0.45	0.19	2.9	0.54	19.0	103.0	0
Soyabean	426	0.73	0.39	3.2	-	8.65	100.0	-
Leafy vegetables								
Amaranth	5,520	0.03	0.30	1.2	-	41.0	149.0	99
Bathua leaves	1,740	0.01	0.14	0.6	-	-	-	35
Brussels sprouts	126	0.05	0.16	0.4	-	-	-	72
Cabbage	120	0.06	0.09	0.4	-	13.3	23.0	124
Coriander leaves	6,918	0.05	0.06	0.8	-	-	-	135
Fenugreek leaves	2,340	0.04	0.31	0.8	-	-	-	52
Lettuce	990	0.09	0.13	0.50	-	-	-	10
Mint	1,620	0.05	0.26	1.0	-	9.7	114.0	27
Mustard leaves	2,622	0.03	-	-	-	-	-	33
Radish leaves	5,295	0.18	0.47	0.8	-	-	-	81
Spinach	5,580	0.03	0.26	0.5	-	51.0	123.0	28

Foodstuff	Carotene (µg)	Thiamin (mg)	Riboflavin (mg)	Niacin (mg)	Vitamin B_6 (mg)	Folic acid(µg) Free	Folic acid(µg) Total	Vitamin C (mg)
Roots and tubers								
Beet root	0	0.04	0.09	0.4	-	-	-	10
Carrot	1,890	0.04	0.02	0.6	-	5.0	15.0	3
Colocasia	24	0.09	0.03	0.4	-	16.0	54.0	0
Onion	15	0.08	0.02	0.5	-	-	-	2
Potato	24	0.10	0.01	1.2	-	3.0	7.0	17
Radish, white	3	0.06	0.02	0.5	-	-	-	15
Sweet potato	6	0.08	0.04	0.7	-	-	-	24
Tapioca	-	0.05	0.10	0.3	-	-	-	25
Turnip	0	0.04	0.04	0.5	-	-	-	43
Yam	78	0.07	-	07	-	0.9	17.5	-
Other vegetables								
Ash gourd	0	0.06	0.01	0.4	-	-	-	1
Bitter gourd	126	0.07	0.09	0.5	-	-	-	88
Bottle gourd	0	0.03	0.01	0.2	-	-	-	0
Brinjal	74	0.04	0.11	0.9	-	5.0	34.0	1
Cauliflower	30	0.04	0.10	10	-	-	-	56
Cucumber	0	0.03	0	0.2	-	12.6	14.7	7
Drumstick	110	0.05	0.07	0.2	-	-	-	120
French bean	132	0.08	0.06	0.3	-	15.5	45.5	24
Ghosala	120	0.02	0.06	0.4	-	-	-	0
Capsicum	427	0.55	0.05	0.1	-	-	-	137
Lady finger	52	0.07	0.10	0.6	-	25.3	105.1	13
Lotus stem, dry	0	0.82	1.21	1.9	-	-	-	3
Plantain, green	30	0.05	0.02	0.3	-	1.6	16.4	24
Pumpkin	50	0.06	0.04	0.5	-	3.0	13.0	2
Ridge gourd	33	-	0.01	0.2	-	-	-	5
Tinda, tender	13	0.04	0.08	0.3	-	-	-	18
Water chestnut, fresh	12	0.05	0.07	0.6	-	-	-	9
Nuts and oilseeds								
Almond	0	0.24	0.57	4.4	-	-	-	0
Cashew nut	60	0.63	0.19	1.2	-	-	-	0
Chilgoza	-	0.32	0.30	3.6	-	-	-	0
Coconut, dry	0	0.08	0.01	3.0	-	15.3	16.5	7
Coconut, fresh	0	0.05	0.10	0.8	-	11.7	12.5	1
Gingelly seeds	60	1.01	0.34	4.4	-	51.0	134.0	0
Groundnut	37	0.90	0.13	19.9	-	16.0	20.0	0
Groundnut, roasted	0	0.39	0.13	22.1	-	-	-	0
Pistachio nut	144	0.67	0.28	2.3	-	-	-	-
Walnut	6	0.45	0,40	1.0	-	-	-	0
Fruits								
Amla	9	0.03	0.01	0.2	-	-	-	600
Apple	0	-	-	0	-	-	-	1
Apricot, fresh	2160	0.04	0.13	0.6	-	-	-	6
Banana, ripe	78	0.05	0.08	0.5	-	-	-	7
Cherries	0	0.08	0.08	0.3	-	-	-	7
Dates, dried	26	0.01	0.02	0.9	-	-	-	3

Foodstuff	Carotene (µg)	Thiamin (mg)	Riboflavin (mg)	Niacin (mg)	Vitamin B₆ (mg)	Folic acid(µg) Free	Folic acid(µg) Total	Vitamin C (mg)
Grapes, pale green	0	-	-	0	-	-	-	1
Guava	0	0.03	0.03	0.4	-	-	-	212
Jack fruit	175	0.03	0.13	0.4	-	-	-	7
Lemon	0	0.02	0.01	0.1	-	-	-	39
Litchi	0	0.02	0.06	0.4	-	-	-	31
Lime, sweet (malta)	0	-	-	0	-	-	-	54
Lime, sweet (mausambi)	0	-	-	0	-	-	-	50
Loquat	559	-	-	0	-	-	-	0
Mango, ripe	2,743	0.08	0.09	0.9	-	-	-	16
Musk melon	169	0.11	0.08	0.3	-	-	-	26
Water melon	0	0.02	0.04	0.1	-	-	-	1
Orange	1,104	-	-	-	-	-	-	30
Orange juice	15	0.06	0.02	0.4	-	-	-	64
Papaya, ripe	666	0.04	0.25	0.2	-	-	-	57
Peaches	0	0.02	0.03	0.5	-	-	-	6
Pears	28	0.06	0.03	0.2	-	-	-	0
Phalsa	419	-	-	0.3	-	-	-	22
Pineapple	18	0.20	0.12	0.1	-	-	-	39
Plum	166	0.04	0.1	0.3	-	-	-	5
Pomegranate	0	0.06	0.10	0.3	-	-	-	16
Raisins	2.4	0.07	0.19	0.7	-	-	-	1
Raspberry	1,248	-	-	0.8	-	-	-	30
Sapota	97	0.02	0.03	0.2	-	-	-	6
Pumpkin	0	0.07	0.17	1.3	-	-	-	37
Strawberry	18	0.03	0.02	2.1	-	-	-	52
Tomato, ripe	351	0.12	0.06	0.4	-	14.0	30.0	27
Fish and other sea foods	Retinol							
Crab, mussel	780	-	-	3.1	-	-	-	-
Hilsa	-	-	-	2.8	-	-	-	24
Katla	-	-	-	0.8	-	-	-	-
Mrigal	-	-	-	0.7	-	9.7	16.7	-
Pomfret, white	-	-	0.15	2.6	-	-	-	-
Prawn	0	0.01	0.10	4.8	-	-	-	-
Rohu	-	0.05	0.07	0.7	-	-	-	22
Sardine	-	-	-	2.6	-	-	-	-
Seer	-	-	-	1.2	-	-	-	-
Shrimp (dried)	-	-	-	-	-	15.7	18.6	-
Meat and poultry	Retinol							
Egg, hen	420	0.10	0.40	0.1	-	70.3	78.3	0
Fowl	-	-	0.14	-	-	3.2	6.8	-
Goat meat (lean)	-	-	-	-	-	0.5	4.5	-
Liver, sheep	6,690	0.36	1.70	17.6	-	65.5	188.8	20
Mutton, muscle	9	0.18	0.14	6.8	-	1.0	5.8	-
Pork, muscle	0	0.54	0.09	2.8	-	-	-	2

Foodstuff	Carotene (µg)	Thiamin (mg)	Riboflavin (mg)	Niacin (mg)	Vitamin B_6 (mg)	Folic acid(µg)		Vitamin C (mg)
						Free	Total	
Milk and milk Products	Retinol							
Milk (buffalo's)	48	0.04	0.10	0.1	-	3.3	5.6	1
Milk (cow's)	53	0.05	0.19	0.1	-	5.6	8.5	2
Milk (human)	41	0.02	0.02	-	-	1.3	-	3
Curd (cow's milk)	31	0.05	0.16	0.1	-	3.3	12.5	1
Skimmed milk, liquid	-	-	-	0.1	-	-	-	1
Chenna (cow's milk)	110	0.07	0.02	-	-	-	-	3
Cheese	82	-	-	-	-	-	-	-
Khoa (cow's milk, full cream)	149	0.23	0.41	0.4	-	-	-	6
Fats and edible oils	Retinol							
Butter	960	-	-	-	-	-	-	-
Ghee (cow)	600	-	-	-	-	-	-	-
Hydrogenated oil, fortified	750	-	-	-	-	-	-	-